GENE ACTION

GENE ACTION

A

Historical

Account

WERNER MAAS

Department of Microbiology
New York University School of Medicine
New York, New York

OXFORD
UNIVERSITY PRESS
2001

OXFORD
UNIVERSITY PRESS

Oxford   New York
Athens   Auckland   Bangkok   Bogotá   Buenos Aires   Calcutta
Cape Town   Chennai   Dar es Salaam   Delhi   Florence   Hong Kong   Istanbul
Karachi   Kuala Lumpur   Madrid   Melbourne   Mexico City   Mumbai
Nairobi   Paris   São Paulo   Shanghai   Singapore   Taipei   Tokyo   Toronto   Warsaw

and associated companies in
Berlin   Ibadan

Copyright © 2001 by Oxford University Press, Inc.

Published by Oxford University Press, Inc.,
198 Madison Avenue, New York, New York, 10016
http://www.oup-usa.org

Library of Congress Cataloging-in-Publication Data
Maas, Werner Karl, 1921–
Gene action : a historical account /
Werner Maas.
p. cm.
Includes bibliographical references.
ISBN 0-19-514131-8
1. Genetics—History. I. Title.
QH428.M33   2001
576.5′09—dc21   00-032417

2 4 6 8 9 7 5 3 1

Printed in the United States of America
on acid-free paper

This book is dedicated to
my wife, Renata Maas,
who firmly believes that
well-reasoned experiments will
lead to the truth.

PREFACE

THE science of genetics was born with the epoch-making experiments of Gregor Mendel during the middle of the nineteenth century. He carried out crosses with pairs of pea plants, with the two members of each pair differing in a single characteristic. From the analysis of many such crosses that were carried out over a 10-year period, he concluded that there were separate determinants for each of the seven traits he was investigating. He named these determinants *elements;* later they were called *genes.* He assumed that the elements of the parents were transmitted through the pollen and eggs and that they were united in the offspring. This theoretical picture of Mendel provided, for the first time, a clear concept of the transfer of genetic information and the expression of this information in the progeny.

The subsequent history of genetics has been divided into two distinct periods. The first, from the time of Mendel until 1940, has been called the Classical Period. During this time it was shown that genes are located in chromosomes and that the Mendelian pattern of inheritance parallels the behavior of chromosomes during reproduction. Changes in individual genes, called gene mutations, made it possible, by crossing mutated plants with their normal parents, to map the position of genes in the chromosomes. The second period, which started in 1940 and is still going on, has been called the period of Molecular Genetics. It originated from the fusion of genetics with biochemistry and it is concerned mainly with the chemical basis of heredity: chemical characterization of genes and the biochemical mechanisms underlying their action.

In the present book I give an account of the history of gene action. To the extent that it is necessary to understand the action of genes, I also include the history of the identification of genes as DNA and the double-helical structure of DNA. The story of DNA has been frequently described and has become a familiar subject. The history of gene action, however, is less well-known and, with the present-day interest in the functions of genes, my account provides useful background knowledge. The high point of my story is the period between 1940 and 1965 when the fundamental features of gene action were discovered.

By a fortunate coincidence I became interested in the gene action problem in 1941, the year in which molecular genetics was launched. I had entered Harvard College in 1939. In high school, I had developed an interest in biology and I decided to major in this subject. After taking introductory courses in General Biology and Comparative Anatomy during the first 2 years, I took genetics in 1941. This course opened a totally new aspect of biology to me, of whose existence I had not been aware. Previous courses had been mostly descriptive without much underlying theory, except for the theory of evolution. In contrast, here I encountered abstract units of inheritance called genes, analogous to molecules in chemistry. They could be treated quantitatively and their transmission from one generation to the next was governed by rules that permitted one to predict the frequencies of different types of offspring. To me, biology became a real science, like chemistry and physics.

There was, however, one feature of the genetics course that bothered me. Why was nothing said about the chemical nature of genes and of their actions? At this time I was also taking a course in biochemistry and was impressed with the beautiful analysis of metabolic pathways described by my inspiring teacher, George Wald. The pathways he discussed were involved in the production of energy, generated in fermentations and oxidations, and its utilization in muscle contraction. Why were such studies not carried out with the activities of genes? I came under the impression that biochemists had never heard of genes and geneticists had never heard of enzymatically controlled reaction steps. At this point I was inspired to investigate the biochemical basis of gene action.

The person who bridged the gap between genetics and biochemistry was George Beadle. In 1940 he was well-known as a maize geneticist and as the coauthor of a textbook of genetics. In the course of his studies he realized that the organisms chosen for genetic studies, such as fruit flies and maize, were unsuitable for biochemistry and that vice versa, organisms used by biochemists, such as rats and pigeons, were not amenable to genetic analysis of biochemical pathways. This realization induced him to look for an organism that combined features suitable for both genetic and biochemcial research. He found it in a microorganism, the bread mold *Neurospora*. Together with his colleague, the biochemist Edward Tatum, he carried out experiments that launched the field of biochemical genetics, later known as molecular genetics.

Looking back now on the history of gene action, starting with the work of Beadle and Tatum, I can discern three well-defined phases during which the major advances in the field occurred. There is the first phase between 1941 and 1953, which led to the realization that the action of a gene involves the determination of the structure of a specific protein molecule. This was formulated by Beadle as the One Gene–One Enzyme hypothesis. During this period there also occurred the identification of DNA as the genetic material.

Following the elucidation of the structure of DNA in 1953, it became possible to envisage concrete mechanisms for the action of genes in determining the structure of protein molecules. To solve this problem required detailed knowledge of the biochemical steps in protein synthesis. This stimulated a great deal of research. Between 1953 and 1961, the second phase, the steps between genes in DNA and their protein products were worked out. The overall scheme was expressed by Francis Crick in the Central Dogma: DNA → RNA → Protein. A code was proposed for utilizing the information contained in DNA for the construction of protein molecules. In 1961, this Genetic Code was deciphered by biochemists.

The third phase in the history of gene action, which overlaps the second phase, started in 1955 with the recognition of special proteins whose sole function was to regulate the activity of genes. This discovery lent a new dimension to our concept of gene action. The genes that controlled the production of regulatory proteins were named regulatory genes. Extensive studies were carried out on the mechanism by which regulatory proteins control gene expression. A model was proposed in 1961, called the Operon Model that combined the known features of the action of genes and their regulation. By 1965, the Operon Model, modified in some details, provided a complete framework for understanding gene action and its regulation.

The major portion of my book, Parts II, III, and IV, deal with the three phases of molecular genetics between 1941 and 1965. I have, in addition, included two sections, Parts I and V. Part I deals with the studies during the Classical Period, in which the foundations were laid for the major emergence of molecular genetics. Part V describes the spectacular advances since 1965 that have led to the present-day pervasive influence of genes and their actions.

My historical account is based largely on my own recollections, implemented by reading accounts written by people I have known. I have also added some of my own work, as it entered into the mainstream of the history of gene action. For Part I, I have relied heavily on the books *History of Genetics* by A.H. Sturtevant and *A Short History of Genetics* by L.C. Dunn. I met Sturtevant in 1946 when I was a postdoctoral fellow at the California Institute of Technology and had several interesting conversations with him. Dunn was one of my advisors when I was a graduate student at Columbia University from 1943 to 1946. I had great admiration for him as a scientist and as a person. In the Appendix, I have listed books and articles that I have used in writing my account.

In the Introduction to his book, written in 1965, Dunn says that, "there must be added at some future time a chapter on the history of molecular genetics." This is the task I have set myself and I am building the history of molecular genetics on top of what Dunn called the history of organismal genetics. In my mind's eye I can see Dunn as he listens to my plan and, in my wishful thinking, I see a nod of approval.

New York, N.Y.
April 2000

W. K. M.

ACKNOWLEDGMENTS

THE idea for writing this book originated during a course I gave on the History of Molecular Genetics at the University of Kaiserslautern in 1992. I thank Timm Anke for giving me the opportunity to teach this course. I also thank Norman Horowitz and my wife, Renata Maas, for critically reading the manuscript and making many helpful suggestions. I am especially grateful to Lynn Koch for her untiring devotion in typing the numerous versions of the manuscript. Finally, I am most grateful to Jeffrey House for steering me in the right direction during the writing of this book.

CONTENTS

I

THE CLASSICAL PERIOD, 1860–1940

G ENETICS as an active field of science actually started in 1900 with the rediscovery of Mendel's publication of 1866. The period during which Mendel carried out his fundamental work, between 1856 and 1870, laying down the principles of the science of genetics, looks like a historical mirage that had broken, as a bright new scientific approach, into the darkness of previous guesses and speculations, only to disappear again and remain buried for 35 years. It took the discovery of chromosomes and their behavior, during this interval, to recognize the significance of Mendel's findings.

The main efforts during the Classical Period were directed toward correlating the behavior of genes, as determined by the method of genetic analysis invented by Mendel, with the behavior of chromosomes during reproduction, as determined by direct microscopic observation. The ratios of offspring that Mendel found were explained by the segregation of paternal and maternal chromosomes in the germ cells prior to their union during fertilization. Detailed genetic studies led to the mapping of genes in the chromosomes. These studies were greatly expanded through the discovery of mutagenic agents, such as X-rays, which made it possible to isolate mutants in many genes. By the end of the Classical Period a complete picture had emerged of the chromosomal mechanics of inheritance.

The majority of geneticists during the Classical Period showed little interest in the chemical nature of genes or the biochemistry of gene action. They felt that genes as units of inheritance were sufficient for the creation of the science of genetics. The successes that were achieved in genetic research and its application to agriculture and medicine justified this attitude. In addition, genetics created a superb scaffold for later biochemical studies, even though it considered genes only as black boxes.

1

Overture:

The Garden of Mendel

M ENDEL carried out his experiments with peas in the garden of the Augustinian Monastery in Brno in the Czech Republic. At the time of his experiments the city was called Brünn and was part of the Habsburg Empire. Brno is the capital of the province of Moravia and is the second-largest city in the Czech Republic. It is 2 hours from Vienna by train.

At the start of the nineteenth century, Brno became the center of the textile industry of the Habsburg Empire. In the area surrounding the city there was much sheep breeding to improve the quality of the wool. The economic advantages of using hybridization in sheep breeding stimulated interest among the farmers in applying hybridization to plant breeding practices, mainly for fruit trees, grapes, and cereals. With an eye to these developments, learned societies were organized, such as an Agricultural Society, an Association of Friends, Experts and Supporters of Sheep Breeding, and a Pomological and Oenological Association. In 1820, G.C.L. Hempel, an expert plant breeder, stated in an article that "higher scientific pomology" (raising of apples) was moving toward the point where the breeder would be able to create a new variety according to a previously conceived ideal type, combining favorable traits of fruit size, shape, color, and flavor. But he emphasized that it first would be necessary to explain the laws of hybridization that applied to sexually reproducing plants. He stated that a new type of natural scientist would have to emerge, able to perform demanding experiments in plant hybridization. He characterized him as "a researcher with a profound knowledge of botany and sharply defined powers of observation, who might, with untiring and stubborn patience, grasp the subtleties of these experiments, take a firm command of them, and provide a clear explanation." This was a prescient description of Mendel, born 2 years later in the village of Hyncice (Heinsdorf) in Moravia.

The Augustinian Monastery became the center of the scientific activities concerned with animal and plant breading with the appointment of C.F. Napp as its abbot in 1824. Napp had a deep interest in these subjects and was an energetic organizer in furthering education and research. He became a widely recognized public figure and exerted great influence, beyond the monastery walls, on the establishment of scientific societies and educational institutions. Besides that, he appreciated high intellectual standards and he assembled around him a group of unusual monks. They had in common an independent and liberal spirit. To illustrate this point, there was a report sent to the Archbishop in Prague by the Bishop of Brno in 1854 after an inspection of the monastery, during which he had spoken to all the monks individually. In it he stated that Abbot Napp held so many public offices that he was unable to devote sufficient attention to his main responsibility, that of running the monastery. As a result, the last ray of spiritual life had faded there. The bishop saw the scientific and teaching activities of the monks as being in contradiction to their spiritual calling. After giving devastating reports on individual monks, he complained that not a single member of the community was willing to admit the error of his ways, and that they stood behind their misguided superior to a man. They had the nerve to ask for a change in the rules of the monastery that would allow them to devote even more time to science and teaching. He recommended that the monastery be dissolved by papal decree. Luckily, Napp, through his wide connections and diplomatic skills, was able to avoid this disaster.

Gregor Mendel entered the Augustinian Monastery in 1843. He was born Johann Mendel, in 1822 into a farming family of German origin. His father grew fruit trees around the house and he introduced his son to the art of grafting at an early age. They were a poor family, especially since during this late feudal period of the Habsburg Empire, the father was obliged to work 3 days a week for his landlord. Johann was sent to the local school and there his teacher noticed that he was a gifted student. On his teacher's advice the parents sent him to a Gymnasium (a secondary school) in a nearby town, although it was a considerable financial hardship. He graduated from the Gymnasium in 1840. During the last 2 years his father, due to an injury, was unable to send him money and Johann supported himself solely by tutoring other students. He wanted to enter a university but to do this he had to spend 2 preparatory years at an institution of higher learning. He did this at the Philosophy Institute at

Olomouc, an old university town, under the most trying circumstances. It was there that his physics professor F. Franz, who was aware of his dire circumstances and had recognized his talents, suggested to him that he should apply for admission to the Augustinian Monastery. Johann followed this advice and, with the help of an enthusiastic recommendation from Franz to Abbot Napp, he was accepted as a novice, the only one of 14 applicants. On entering the monastery he adopted Gregor as his first name.

During the first few years at the monastery, Mendel studied philosophy and theology and carried out his spiritual duties, such as caring for the sick at a hospital. The latter activity upset him. Abbot Napp, seeing his distress, relieved him of this duty and instead arranged for him to teach parttime at a secondary school in Znojmo, a nearby town. There he taught mathematics and Greek in the seventh grade. This gave him much pleasure. In order to become a fulltime teacher, he had to pass an examination that was administered by a group of professors at the University of Vienna. Mendel took this examination and failed it. This was a great disappointment to him, but in the long run it turned out to be a blessing in disguise.

In 1851, Mendel substituted for a short time as a teacher of Natural History at the Brno Technical School, which later became a university. He received high praise from the headmaster who considered him to be a first-rate teacher in every respect. Clearly his failure in the examinations in Vienna was not taken seriously in Brno. At that time Abbot Napp arranged for Mendel to go to Vienna for further scientific training at the University. Napp had sent a letter to the Bishop of Brno, stating that "Father Gregor Mendel had proved unsuitable for work as a parish priest, but had on the other hand shown evidence of exceptional intellectual capacity and remarkable industry in the natural sciences."

At the age of 29 years Mendel now had a chance to complete his education at a university. Had he passed his teacher's examination, he would have stayed on at the Znojmo Gymnasium, and several generations of secondary school students would have gained an excellent teacher. Science, on the other hand, would almost certainly have lost one of its great discoverers.

Mendel spent 2 years, from 1851 to 1853, at the University of Vienna. His main fields of study were physics and botany. One of his professors in physics was Christian Doppler (of the Doppler effect). Doppler had published a textbook on arithmetic and algebra in which he outlined the principles of combinatorial theory and the theory of probability in relation to the needs of applied science. Besides learning from Doppler theories of physics and skills required to perform experiments, he profited greatly from the mathematical treatment of probability in Doppler's textbook for his later work on plant hybridization. Doppler died in 1853. His successor, A. Ettingshausen, also emphasized the use of mathematics in the study of physics. He had published a textbook on Combinatorial Analysis and two volumes of lectures in higher mathematics.

Mendel continued his studies with him and this contributed more to his mathematical education.

His professor in botany was Franz Unger, an outstanding plant physiologist. Unger was strongly influenced by J.M. Schleiden, one of the originators of the Cell Theory. Schleiden stated that he was offering a guide to a new manner of plant research. He was sure that botanists lacked an essential knowledge of chemistry and physics, without which the "real development of the science of organisms" was unimaginable. Unger had a very broad approach to botany, including paleobotany and the evolution of plants, environmental effects on plant development, and hybridization to produce new varieties. He was re- garded highly among natural scientists. When a new Natural Science Society was founded in Brno, Unger was among the first 24 honorary members. The contact with Unger as a teacher left a strong impression on Mendel.

After his return from Vienna, Mendel started to plan his experiments on plant hybridization. He also resumed his activities as a teacher, this time at the Realschule, a new technically oriented secondary school in Brno. This school had acquired a distinguished faculty. An outstanding member was A. Zawadski, who had recently been deprived of his professorial chair at Lemberg (now Lwoff) in the Ukraine. The authorities in Vienna had held him responsible for the student unrest in 1848, and he was obliged to leave not only the university but also the city. Mendel, in his new position, taught physics and natural sci- ence. He had frequent contacts with Zawadski. He soon became a very popular teacher and continued in this position for many years.

In 1855, Mendel applied once more to take the teacher's examination. Al- most ironically, he failed again, this time because of a conflict with one of his examiners, Professor E. Fenzl. Apparently Fenzl believed that plant embryos arose from the male pollen tube and the female germ cell was only responsible for its nutrition. Mendel believed that both parental germ cells contributed to the inherited traits of the embryo. Mendel's view turned out to be correct.

For his experiments on hybridization, Mendel chose to work on garden peas. There were many varieties available that were easy to grow. When crossed with each other, they produced fertile hybrids that could be propagated farther, either by self-fertilization or by cross-fertilization. Mendel chose seven pairs among the available varieties that could be distinguished by a clearly recogniz- able trait. For example, one pair differed in the shape of the ripe seeds: either round or wrinkled; another pair differed in the length of the stem: either tall or short; another pair differed in the color of the ripe seeds: either green or yel- low. He bred these varieties for 2 years before starting his crosses to be sure that they bred true. Once he was sure that the traits were stably inherited, he crossed the two members of each pair with each other. He found that the first- generation offspring were all of one kind, resembling one of the parents. For example, in the cross of tall versus short plants, the offspring were all tall.

When these plants were self-fertilized, they produced two kinds of off-spring, tall and short. When Mendel counted the offspring, he found that there were three times as many tall plants as there were short plants. When he self-fertilized these plants, the short plants gave rise only to short plants, they bred true. Among the tall plants, one-third gave rise to only tall plants, they bred true like the short plants. The other two-thirds gave rise, like the first generation hybrids, to tall and short plants, again in a ration of three tall to one short.

Over an 8-year period, Mendel carried out the same crossing experiments with all seven pairs and he always obtained the same numerical results, always the 3:1 ratio in the second generation. When he did crosses with pairs in which two traits were combined, such as tall stems and round seeds versus short stems and wrinkled seeds, he obtained the same 3:1 ratio for each pair of traits. Although they were present in the same plant, the two traits were transmitted independently of each other.

Before Mendel had started his experiments there had been other botanists who carried out similar experiments, but Mendel's experiments differed from all previous ones in two important respects: he dealt with single traits, whereas previous experimenters had lumped several differences together; he counted his progeny, obtaining quantitative results, which nobody before him had done. This enabled him to construct a hypothesis that gave a clear explanation of his results. He postulated that each of his seven traits was determined by what he called a separate element. Fifty years later it was called a *gene*. He assumed that each element was present in duplicate. The two were either identical or they were different forms of the same element. For example, the element that determined the shape of the ripe seeds could exist in a form that gave rise to round seeds or alternatively, in a form that gave rise to wrinkled seeds. When the two different elements were present in the same plant, only the element determing round seeds was expressed. Its presence suppressed the expression of the element for wrinkled seeds. Mendel explained this by saying that the expression of the element for round seeds was dominant over the expression of the element for wrinkled seeds. Genetically, plants with round seeds were of two kinds. Either they contained cells with two identical elements for round seeds or one element for round seeds and one element for wrinkled seeds.

In Mendel's time it was known that during fertilization pollen cells united with egg cells to give rise to an embryo. It was generally believed that this occurred in a 1:1 ratio. Mendel assumed that during the formation of egg and pollen cells, the duplicate forms of each element were separated so that the pollen cells and egg cells contained only one copy. The distribution of the different elements after separation was at random. After the fusion of pollen and eggs during fertilization, the elements contributed by each parent came together again and the duplicate number was restored. The joinings of different kinds of pollen and eggs also occurred at random. By making these assumptions of random distribution of elements in the formation of germ cells and in their reunion after fertilization, Mendel's calculations of the expected ratios of offspring agreed with the experimental results he had obtained.

Mendel's hypothesis of the random segregation of genes and their subsequent independent assortment provided a complete picture of the mechanism of inheritance. The details of this mechanism were the main topic of investigation during the Classical Period between 1900 and 1940, when the transmission of genes was linked to the transmission of chromosomes present in the nucleus. The experimental method that Mendel invented for his studies became the standard methodology for genetic analysis. "Mendelism" became the foundation of the Science of Genetics.

Besides Mendel's hypothesis for the transmission of genes, there is another hypothesis of his which is of major importance for the history of gene action, the subject of the present book. This is that each inherited trait is controlled by a single element. This perceptive concept of Mendel marks the beginning of the history of gene action. Its significance was not fully realized until the end of the Classical Period, when biochemistry entered the field. The methodology that Mendel provided to study the action of elements was to compare the effects produced by two different forms of the same element and the interaction between two different elements in the same cell. This methodology has remained to be a powerful tool for the study of gene action. It has been especially useful for dissecting gene-controlled metabolic pathways.

Mendel completed his work on peas in 1865. At that time he presented a summary in two lectures given to the fellow members of the Natural Science Society of Brno. He also published a paper of 47 pages that described all his work in the Proceedings of this society. The lectures were received with polite interest, but nobody in the audience appreciated the significance of what they had heard. The publication was widely distributed, included the mailing out of 40 reprints, but was ignored by the scientific community.

After 1865, Mendel carried out experiments with other plant species and obtained results that were similar to those obtained with peas. It became clear that his hypothesis was of general validity. He entered into a prolonged correspondence with the outstanding botanist Carl Nägeli, whom he had met during his student days in Vienna. Nägeli took interest in Mendel's work and made suggestions for further experiments, but even he did not understand the significance of Mendel's work.

In 1868, Abbot Napp died and Mendel was elected his successor. This change in Mendel's life had disastrous consequences. The work involved in administering the monastery took all his time and he had no time left for scientific work, although he wanted to do science. Mendel was not a diplomatic administrator and was stubborn in maintaining his beliefs. He became embroiled in a controversy with the Austrian government over taxation of monastery property that took a long time and consumed much of his energy. He was involved with various committees and even functioned for a time as the director of a local bank. All these worries and commitments embittered him and finally ruined his health. He died in 1884 at the age of 62.

Mendel was a popular man and many people attended his funeral. They remembered him for many things: his devoted teaching, his kindness helping people in need, his activities as the local meteorologist, his activities as a plant breeder and as a bee keeper. Nobody realized that the world had lost one of the great geniuses of science. After his death, his fellow monks went through his voluminous notes but could not see any use for them and burnt them all.

The question has often been raised of why the significance of Mendel's work was not recognized by his contemporaries. Several different reasons have been given. My own feeling is that Mendel's ideas were novel and did not fit into current thinking about biological problems. Besides, Mendel's mathematical approach was that used by physicists and most biologists were not familiar with it. Under these circumstances the natural reaction of scientists toward a theory they cannot comprehend is to say that it is wrong or to ignore it. Mendel tried to console himself by saying that "my time will come," but 30 years turned out to be too long for him to wait.

2

Building a Scaffold:

Genes Within Chromosomes

B ETWEEN 1865 and 1900 major developments occurred in the study of cells, resulting in a field called cytology. It was in the structure and function of the nucleus where important discoveries were made. It was shown that during part of the life cycle of a cell, material present in the nucleus condensed into thread-like structures called chromosomes. The number of chromosomes was the same in all cells of an organism and was characteristic of the species. Prior to cell division, the chromosomes divided in a process called mitosis and each daughter cell received one complete set of chromosomes. In the formation of the male and female germ cells a reduction occurred in the number of chromosomes. During one cell division, the chromosomes did not divide and their number was reduced to half. This reduction division was later called meiosis. At fertilization, male and female germ cells were united and the full complement of chromosomes was restored. All these observations on mitosis and meiosis were made possible by improved techniques of microscopy and by the development of staining techniques by which chromosomes could be visualized. The word chromosome, introduced in 1885, reflects this technique (chromo = color; soma = body).

Because of the constancy of the number of chromosomes and their equal division during mitosis it seemed likely that they were involved in the transmission of material linked to heredity. This was further borne out by the reduction of the chromosome number to half during meiosis and the restoration of the duplicate set after fertilization. Although the observations that had been made did not *prove* that the nucleus was the physical basis of inheritance, cytologists generally believed that it was a good working hypothesis. The picture that emerged from these studies formed a background for explaining Mendel's laws of heredity but these were forgotten.

The rediscovery of Mendel's work occurred in 1900. Carl Correns in Germany, Erich von Tschermak in Austria, and Hugo de Vries in Holland carried out plant hybridization experiments that produced the same results as those obtained by Mendel. Each thought at first that he had made an original discovery but then became aware of Mendel's paper and found that he had only confirmed work carried out 40 years earlier. The results of the three investigators were published independently in the spring of 1900. This date marks the actual beginning of genetics as a full-blown science.

Correns studied botany and did his doctoral work in 1889 under the guidance of Naegeli, from whom he first heard about Mendel. Subsequently he studied the genetic constitution of the endosperm tissue in maize and in the course of this work carried out hybridizations not only with maize but also with other plant species. In his results he noticed the occurrence of sharp segregation of alternative characters and this led him in 1899 to Mendel's 1866 paper. Correns realized that the explanation he had just reached had been worked out in masterly fashion 33 years earlier. After he rediscovered Mendel's work he made the revealing remark that "whoever supports with his arguments the establishment of a correct view of another person, may have accomplished more than he who first proposed it." Later he became a leading plant geneticist in Germany and as a result was appointed the first director of the newly founded Kaiser Wilhem Institut für Biologie in Berlin-Dahlem. During his tenure there he carried out extensive research but unfortunately most of the records of his work were still unpublished when during the bombing of Berlin in 1945 all of them were destroyed.

Tschermak was primarily interested in practical plant breeding. In the course of his studies he carried out crosses with the same varieties of peas as Mendel had done and obtained the same results. He thus confirmed Mendel's work, although his experiments were much more limited than Mendel's. There is an unwitting connection between him and Mendel in that he was a grandson of Fenzl, under whom Mendel studied systematic botany and microscopy during his stay in Vienna in 1851 and who later was responsible for his failure to become a certified teacher.

The most illustrious of the three rediscoverers was de Vries. He was professor of botany at the University of Amsterdam. He was interested in the nature of the variations that were responsible for Darwinian natural selection and he came to the conclusion that they were much more discrete than the small continuous variations Darwin had proposed. He found and studied his postulated, discontinuous variations (sports) in a bed of evening primroses growing in the wild in Hilversum in Holland where he spent his summer holidays. On the basis of his studies he proposed that it was these discrete changes, which he called mutations, that made evolution by natural selection possible. He announced his Mutationtheorie in 1900, the same year in which he reported his plant breeding studies that had resulted in his resurrection of Mendel's work. He had been led into these latter studies also through his interest in the mechanism of evolution. Not being aware of Mendel's findings he had formulated his own theory of inheritance in which he postulated the existence of independent units of heredity somewhat similar to Mendel's units. He stated that "According to the principles I have expressed, the specific characters of organisms are composed of separate units. One is able to study, experimentally, these units either by the phenomena of variability and mutability or by the production of hybrids." It was in studies on production of hybrids that he reproduced Mendel's results. Thus, in the same year, 1900, de Vries not only opened up the field of genetics, but he also proposed the concept that mutations are the source of the variations responsible for evolution.

Another person who greatly influenced the launching of genetics in 1900, although he was not one of the original rediscoverers of Mendel's paper, was the British zoologist William Bateson. His interest in inheritance was aroused by Professor W.K. Brooks whom he visited at the summer laboratory of Johns Hopkins University at Hampton, Virginia, during 1883 and 1884. Brooks was also the mentor of two of the other giants of genetics, T.H. Morgan and E.B. Wilson. Bateson, like de Vries, had doubts about Darwin's idea of small continuous variations being the raw material of natural selection and began to investigate discrete, discontinuous variations by carrying out hybridizations with cultivated plants. In 1897, he received a grant to do his studies in the Cambridge Botanical Garden. In the course of these he became aware of Mendel's work and welcomed it with enthusiasm.

Bateson's wife has described in her memoirs his first exposure to Mendel as follows: "On May 8, 1900, on the train to London to deliver a lecture at the Royal Horticultural Society, he read Mendel's paper on peas for the first time. As a lecturer he was always cautious, suggesting rather than confirming his own convictions. So ready was he however for the simple Mendelian law that he at once incorporated it into his lecture."

From that day on Bateson became a devotee of what he soon came to call Mendelism. He carried out breeding experiments with both plants and animals to test the general validity of Mendel's Laws. In his voluminous writings he defended the new view of heredity against criticisms by biometricians who thought that the generality of Mendel's conclusions was unlikely. In 1902 he published a monograph entitled, "Mendel's Principles of Heredity, A Defense," which became the first textbook presentation of the elementary facts of genetics. He coined several terms that have become household words, such as *alleles* for the alternative forms of Mendel's elements, *heterozygote* and *homozygote* to denote whether the two forms of an element present in a cell are different or the same, and, in fact, *genetics* for the new science of heredity. In 1909, he published the first textbook of genetics entitled, "Mendel's Principles of Heredity" which gave an account of all the discoveries made by the application of Mendel's method of research. It also contained an English translation of Mendel's papers and a biographical sketch of Mendel. (I acquired a copy of this book during my graduate student days in 1945, when I found it among books discarded by the Free Library of Philadelphia.)

During the decade following the rediscovery of Mendel's work the principles established by him with peas were tested in many plants and animals and were found to be generally valid. For example, Bateson demonstrated Mendelian inheritance in fowl, and the French scientist Lucien Cuénot demonstrated it in mice. Cuénot found that there could be more than two forms of a gene and, thus, introduced the concept of multiple alleles. The physician Archibald Garrod, who knew Bateson, found that certain disorders of human metabolism were inherited in Mendelian fashion. We shall return to these later. Of medical importance was the analysis of the inheritance of human blood groups. Of great commercial importance were the genetic studies on strains of maize that led to the production of high-yielding hybrid corn. Between 1900 and 1910 Mendelian genetics became a very active field of investigation with wide applications.

During this decade, there was also much research done on chromosomes to establish their role as the carriers of the units of inheritance. First it was shown by Theodor Boveri, in 1902, in ingenious experiments with sea urchins that a full complement of the 18 chromosome pairs was necessary for normal development. Boveri concluded from his work that each chromosome had its own individuality. This conclusion was substantiated in the same year by the experiments of Walter Sutton, a student of C.E. McClung (see next paragraph for his contributions) who subsequently became a graduate student of E.B. Wilson at Columbia University. Sutton showed by careful microscopic measurements that the 11 pairs of chromosomes in grasshopper cells are all of different sizes, but the two chromosomes in a pair were the same size. He studied the chromosomes during reduction division in the germ cells and after fusion following fertilization. From his observation he concluded that "the association of paternal and maternal chromosomes in pairs and then subsequent separation during the reducing division may indicate the physical basis of the Mendelian law of heredity." In a brilliant paper published in 1903 entitled "The Chromosomes in Heredity" he elaborated on this conclusion. At that time he was 23 years old. This was the first correlation of observations on chromosomes with the results of experimental breeding. The new field of cytogenetics, resulting from the fusion of cytology and genetics, may be said to have originated with the work of Sutton and Boveri. Sutton never finished his graduate work but received a degree in medicine and became a practicing surgeon. He died in 1916 at the age of 39 without having returned to his original work.

Another major advance was the finding that there were characteristic chromosomes for each sex. The first suggestion of the relation of a particular chromosome to sex determination was made by C.E. McClung in 1901. He postulated that the so-called accessory "X chromosome," first described by H. Henking in 1891 in the male of an insect, is male determining. For a long time it was considered doubtful that it was a chromosome and its uncertain nature was the reason for giving it the designation "X." (Nowadays it is known by this name.) Definitive cytological demonstrations of sex chromosomes in different species were made in 1905 by Nettie Stevens and E.B. Wilson. At that time it was also found that certain inherited traits were confined to only one sex. They were called sex-linked. It was T.H. Morgan, a colleague of E.B. Wilson at Columbia University who first demonstrated the location of sex-linked genes in the X chromosome of the fruit fly *Drosophila melanogaster.*

Morgan had come to the Zoology Department at Columbia University in 1905. His research interests were then in embryology, the study of development from egg to adult. During the end of the decade he started to work with *Drosophila.* He set out to look for mutant flies in his stocks. It was the finding of a white-eyed mutant male fly that initiated his investigations of *Drosophila* genetics. On further crosses with normal red-eyed females he found that the mutation was expressed only in male flies; in other words, it was sex linked. He assumed that the gene was located in the X chromosome. He further inferred from his breeding experiments that female flies carry two X chromosomes, whereas male flies carry only one X chromosome. In the cross with a normal red-eyed female, all the offspring were red-eyed, because they inherited at least one X chromosome from the mother, and the expression of red eye color is dominant over white eye color. By appropriate crosses, Morgan eventually managed to obtain white-eyed females that carried the mutation in both X chromosomes—they were homozygous for the white eye color.

Later, Morgan found another sex-linked mutant in which the body color was yellow. He showed that in crosses the two sex-linked mutations did not segregate freely from each other, but remained linked, as one would expect if they were located in the same chromosome.

Two future associates, Calvin Bridges and Alfred Sturtevant were undergraduates in 1909 when they decided to take a course in zoology. Morgan happened to give the opening lectures in this course, the only time he did this during his 24 years at Columbia. The two students were so impressed by Morgan that they decided to read about his work, including his studies on the white-eyed mutant. They found the work fascinating and wanted to participate in it. Bridges managed to get a job in Morgan's laboratory washing the milk bottles in which flies were raised. Alfred Sturtevant came from an academically inclined family. His older brother Edgar became a professor of linguistics at Yale. A nephew, Julian Sturtevant, became a professor of organic chemistry at Yale. (Many years later, Alfred and Edgar received honorary degrees at the same Yale commencement.) Sturtevant had written an essay on the pedigree of the horses that had been bred on his father's farm in Alabama, which he showed to Morgan. Morgan liked the essay and offered Sturtevant a working space in his laboratory. At about this time Bridges, who had extraordinary powers of observation, noticed a fly that had very bright red eyes in contrast to normal flies, whose eyes are of a dull red color inside a milk bottle. On his own, he bred this fly and found that the bright red color was inherited. He called the mutation vermilion. Morgan was so impressed with Bridges' performance that he also offered him a work space. This was the beginning of a relationship in which Morgan was known as the boss and Sturtevant and Bridges were known as the boys.

A third future associate Herman Muller, who graduated from Columbia College in 1910, had taken a course with E.B. Wilson. He had also read Wilson's book, *The Cell in Development and Inheritance*, which was the bible for biologists interested in cell structures. After his graduation, Muller wanted to join Morgan's laboratory immediately but had to wait 2 years before a place became available. During these 2 years he worked at several places, but kept in close touch with Morgan's work through frequent visits and discussions.

From the beginning the work of Morgan and his students was very successful. Morgan had by then demonstrated, by mating experiments, the association of several mutations with the X chromosome. This was known as genetic linkage. He had noticed that in crosses some of these mutations were separated from each other among the offspring whereas others remained linked together. He called this separation process *crossing over*, indicating that part of one chromosome had been exchanged with the corresponding part of its partner chromosome. He concluded that genes near each other remained linked and that genes far away from each other were separated. Sturtevant had the innovative idea of quantifying these relationships. After tabulating the frequency of different kinds of offspring he devised a simple statistical method for mapping the location of the mutations in the chromosome. This became the general method for mapping genes. Bridges was able to establish a direct correlation between the unexpected behavior of a sex-linked mutant and an attachment between two X chromosomes to each other observed under the microscope. He thus demonstrated directly that sex-linked genes are located on the sex chromosomes. The rapid further progress of their studies culminated in 1915 in the publication of *The Mechanism of Mendelian Heredity* by T.H. Morgan, A.H. Sturtevant, H.J. Muller, and C.B. Bridges. This book interpreted the whole field of Mendelism in terms of chromosomal structure and behavior. It became a milestone in the history of genetics. At this time the Zoology Department of Columbia University had become the stronghold of genetic research.

As the work carried out by the three brilliant young investigators under the tutelage of Morgan became known, it attracted many visiting scientists. The laboratory, known as the Fly Room, was small, 16 by 23 feet. Eight desks were crowded into it for the use of the investigators. They were littered with notebooks, microscopes, and milk bottles used to breed the flies. The smell of bananas, used as fly food, permeated the room. Sturtevant has given the following description of the intellectual atmosphere of this room:

> This group worked as a unit. Each carried on his own experiments, but each knew exactly what the others were doing, and each new result was freely discussed. There was little attention paid to priority or to the source of new ideas or new interpretations. What mattered was to get ahead with the work. There was much to be done; there were many new ideas to be tested, and many new experimental techniques to be developed. There can have been few times and places in scientific laboratories with such an atmosphere of excitement and with such a record of sustained enthusiasm. This was due in large part to Morgan's own attitude, compounded of enthusiasm combined with a strong critical sense, generosity, open-mindedness, and a remarkable sense of humor. No small part of the success of the undertaking was due also to Wilson's unfailing support and appreciation of the work.

After 1915 there were many notable advances in genetics based on the work of the Morgan Group both with *Drosophila* and with other organisms including humans. An outstanding example was the finding by Muller that irradiation with X-rays induces mutations. This was of enormous importance because it made possible the isolation of mutants at will. From a theoretical point of view, it demonstrated that physical agents could alter genes and this implied that genes had a definite physical structure. Muller was awarded a Nobel prize in 1946 for his discovery. Morgan also received a Nobel prize, in 1934, and it has been said that if the present practice of giving this award to several people involved in the same discovery had been in vogue in 1934, Sturtevant and Bridges would surely have shared the Prize with Morgan.

A development that greatly increased the power of cytogenetic analysis was the finding by Theophilus Painter of giant chromosomes in the salivary glands of *Drosophila* and other species of flies. In these large chromosomes darkly staining bands could be discerned whose position could be correlated with the position of genes, as determined by genetic analysis. The construction of salivary maps by Bridges provided an unexpectedly detailed verification of the chromosomal theory of heredity. It was a spectacular confirmation of the ideas about the structure of the genetic system that had been gained from breeding analysis.

Of the work that was done on the genetics of plants, an outstanding example was the research carried out at Cornell University by R.A. Emerson, a friend of Morgan, on the genetics of maize. Emerson attracted a group of unusual young students, similar to those assembled by Morgan, and their work did much to elucidate the genetic constitution and nature of the chromosomes in maize. Two of these students, Barbara McClintock and George Beadle, were later awarded Nobel prizes.

Around 1940, the period of Classical Genetics drew to a close. It had established that there were traits that were inherited separately and that their transmission followed definite rules. These traits were determined by units called genes that are located in the chromosomes. There were many genes in each chromosome. During reproduction, genes were shuffled, like cards in a deck, either by the independent assortment of chromosomes or by crossing over between regions within homologous chromosomes at meiosis. Genetic changes occurred as a result of mutations within genes or of chromosomal aberrations, involving blocks of adjacent genes. It was the genetic differences created by mutations that made it possible to carry out what is called genetic analysis, as established by Mendel.

During the Classical Period, geneticists were occupied mostly with the physical location and transmission of genes and they did not pay much attention to the question of their chemical constitution or mode of action. As stated by Morgan in his Nobel lecture in 1934: "What are genes? Now that we locate them in the chromosomes are we justified in regarding them as material units; as chemical bodies of a higher order than molecules? Frankly, these are questions with which the working geneticist has not much concerned himself . . . At the level at which the genetic experiments lie, it does not make the slightest difference whether the gene is a hypothetical unit or whether the gene is a material particle. In either case the unit is associated with a specific chromosome, and can be localized there by purely genetic analysis."

During the Classical Period there were major advances in the chemistry of the nucleus, although geneticists did not pay too much attention to them. I shall give a brief account of them because they were important for the developments that occurred during the following period of Molecular Genetics.

The biochemical investigations began in 1869 with the work of Friedrich Miescher. After receiving an MD degree in 1868 from the University of Basel, Switzerland, he decided to do research on the chemistry of physiological processes. This idea had become popular during the middle of the nineteenth century, mainly with the work of Claude Bernard in France and Rudolf Virchow in Germany. Miescher reasoned that the material basis of heredity must lie within the nuclei of living cells, and that the most important of all biochemical tasks was to isolate and characterize these substances. To do this he went to the laboratory of Felix Hoppe-Seyler in Tübingen, Germany, and there started to work on the nuclei of pus cells, a material that was abundantly available at that time in a clinical setting.

Soon after his arrival, Miescher extracted from pus cells a nonprotein, acid material rich in phosphorus. Nothing like it had been described before. Based on its source, Miescher called the new material *nuclein*. Later, in 1889, it was renamed *nucleic acid*.

Miescher's work on the nuclein of pus cells was a prelude to his most important biochemical investigations during 1871–1873 after his return to his native Basel. There he carried out extensive studies on the nuclein isolated from the sperm of the Rhine salmon. Basel was suitable for such research, as it was the center of the salmon fishing industry. Salmon that travel up the Rhine during the spawning season are a rich source of gonadal tissue. Sperm heads are essentially equivalent to cell nuclei and this made salmon sperm an ideal material for Miescher's studies. He carried out chemical analyses of the nucleic acids and also identified a basic protein associated with nucleic acid, which he named protamine.

Toward the end of the nineteenth century, Miescher's work attracted the attention of cytologists and the notion became prevalent that nuclein was the principal material of the recently discovered chromosomes and the very stuff of heredity. As E.B. Wilson stated in 1895: "Now chromatin [the material of chromosomes] is known to be similar to, if not identical with, a substance known as nuclein . . . And thus we reach the remarkable conclusion that inheritance may perhaps be effected by the physical transmission of a particular chemical compound (nuclein) from parent to offspring."

Unfortunately, after these promising beginnings, further studies on the chemistry of nucleic acids led to a change in the opinion of cytologists and, later, geneticists. This change was due to some erroneous notions about nucleic acids that made their role as the hereditary material unlikely. As a result, it became to be accepted that proteins, rather than nucleic acids, fulfilled this role. A statement by E. B. Wilson in 1925 reflects this change: "A large and increasing body of evidence shows that some of the proteins differ characteristically from species to species, and even indicate that they may constitute the fundamental chemical basis of heredity." Unfortunately this change in attitude very much delayed the recognition of Miescher's discovery and, as in the case of Mendel, there was a period of many years, lasting until 1945, before the significance of his findings was fully appreciated. In a letter written shortly before his death in 1895, Miescher stated that the questions relating to the physical basis of heredity will be "fought out between the morphologists and the biochemists during the twentieth century." Boveri, in noting this remark, added that "the biochemist Miescher's entire lifework expressed sufficiently clearly the conviction that the victory will go to his field . . . He (Boveri) himself could think of nothing better than the possibility that morphological analysis would lead to a point where the final elements are chemical compounds."

The successor to Miescher in the study of nucleic acids was Albrecht Kossel. He, like Miescher, started his research career in Hoppe-Seyler's laboratory and from there went to Basel. In later years he held positions in Berlin, Marburg, and Heidelberg, where he carried out his many studies on nucleic acids and nuclear proteins. In 1910 he was awarded a Nobel Prize. Kossel's chief contribution in the nucleic acid field was the isolation and identification of the nucleic acid bases. These were the purines adenine and guanine and the pyrimidines cytosine, thymine (in calf thymus nucleic acid), and uracil (in yeast nucleic acid). He also noted the presence of a 5-carbon sugar in all nucleic acids.

Following Kossel, the most important investigations on the chemistry of nucleic acids were carried out by Phoebus Aaron Levene at the newly established Rockefeller Institute for Medical Research in New York City. Levene had studied in Borodin's Chemical Institute in St. Petersburg in Russia before coming to the United States in 1891. (Borodin was a Professor of Chemistry as well as a composer.) At the beginning of the twentieth century Levene was invited to join the staff of the Rockefeller Institute.

Levene identified the 5-carbon sugar in yeast nucleic acid as D-ribose and the 5-carbon sugar in calf thymus nucleic acid as 2-deoxy-D-ribose. He showed that these sugars were joined at one end to a nucleic acid base and at the other to a phosphate. Such a base–sugar–phosphate compound was called a nucleotide. Since he found that the four bases were present in equal amounts, he postulated that a nucleic acid molecule consists of four nucleotides linked to each other and containing the four different bases in a specified order. This became known as the tetranucleotide hypothesis.

At this point, two kinds of nucleic acid had been recognized, one with D-ribose and uracil in yeast and the other with deoxy-D-ribose and thymine in calf thymus. Because of their source they were denoted as animal nucleic acid and plant nucleic acid. Later, in 1924, when a stain became available, called the Feulgen stain, that gave a color with thymus nucleic acid but not with yeast nucleic acid, the division between plant and animal nucleic acid was shown to be erroneous. They were renamed ribonucleic acid (RNA) and deoxyribonucleic (DNA) acid on the basis of their sugar component. It was shown that RNA and DNA were present in both animal tissues and plant tissues; DNA was in the nucleus and RNA was in the cytoplasm.

At the same time Einar Hammersten in Sweden used a very gentle method for isolating nucleic acids and found that the molecules isolated by him were much larger than the previously isolated molecules and, in fact, the postulated tetranucleotide molecules. This put the tetranucleotide hypothesis in doubt, unless one assumed that Hammersten's macromolecules were composed of blocks of tetranucleotides linked together.

At this point it becomes pertinent to ask why the notion of nucleic acid being the gene-containing hereditary substance was abandoned in favor of proteins. The main reason was an absence of variation in the tetranucleotide structure that could account for genetic differences. The presumed monotony of the nucleic acid structure became a block against accepting nucleic acids as the carriers of genetic information. This block persisted into the 1940s until finally the validity of the tetranucleotide hypothesis began to be questioned. In 1946, the biochemist John Masson Gulland pointed out that there was no indisputable evidence that nucleotides are arranged in other than a random manner in nucleic acid macromolecules. This would permit an immense number of variations in these molecules in contrast to Levene's tetranucleotide structure, which permitted no variation at all.

Prior to Gulland's comment there had been a firm belief that genes consisted of proteins, perhaps nucleoproteins. Moreover, their structure and actions were very complicated and would take many years to disentangle. After his comments, the situation changed and nucleic acids began to be considered seriously as candidates for being the genetic material.

II

ONE GENE–
ONE ENZYME,
1900–1953

Do not discard a hypothesis because it is simple—it might be right.

George W. Beadle

DURING the period covered in Part II, the main outcome of studies on gene action was that each gene controls the formation of a specific enzyme. Enzymes are proteins that catalyze reactions in all cellular functions. During the Classical Period, the evidence for this view of gene action was sporadic, but beginning with the Period of Molecular Genetics in 1940 it became a central focus for research projects.

There were three reasons for this sudden upswing in studies on gene action in 1940.

The first was the introduction of microorganisms into genetic studies. It was already known in 1940 that fungi contain genes that are analogous to the genes of higher forms, such as *Drosophila* and man. The same was demonstrated for bacteria later, in the mid-1940s. Microorganisms are much more amenable to a biochemical approach than higher forms and therefore make it more feasible to study the action of genes in the control of metabolism at the chemical level.

The second was the advances in biochemistry, both in regard to methods for studying metabolic reactions and in regard to general knowledge. For example it was not certain until the end of the 1920s that enzymes are proteins, although the existence of enzymes as organic catalysts had been known since the middle of the nineteenth century.

21

The third was the realization that the basic metabolic processes in the utilization of nutrients and the synthesis of cellular constituents were similar in microorganisms and higher organisms. This led to the concept of the Unity of Biochemistry, which meant that information gained from studies with microorganisms could be applied to higher organisms.

In the 1940s geneticists and biochemists were for the most part still far apart from each other. This hampered the emergence of the new field of biochemical genetics. However, the realization that genes control the production of enzymes, as well as other proteins, began to promote the breakdown of this barrier and laid the foundation for the spectacular advances of the 1950s and 1960s.

3

The Dawn of the One Gene–
One Enzyme Hypothesis
During the Classical Period

WE have seen that during the Classical Period geneticists occupied themselves mainly with working out the mechanism of gene transmission from one generation to the next. Yet many of them could not resist speculating about the way in which genes produce specific effects on the appearance of organisms. Since enzymes were known to be specific catalysts in cellular metabolism, these speculations usually ended up with the involvement of enzymes. In surveying the literature I found the names of 17 geneticists who implicated enzymes in gene action. Some of them, such as Bateson, Muller, and Cuénot, are encountered in the Chapter 2.

A favorite trait studied by geneticists of the Classical Period was pigmentation. The study of inherited color patterns in plants and animals provides aesthetic enjoyment, and because the chemistry of these pigments was beginning to be known in the early 1900s, there was the possibility of analyzing the chemistry underlying genetic differences. For example, Cuénot, who as we have seen established Mendelian inheritance in mice as early as 1903, proposed gene action via enzymes. He assumed that the difference between the gray mice and the black mice he was studying was due to the absence of an enzyme in the black mice. He postulated three active genes in the gray mice, one for a precursor of pigment and two for enzymes that convert the precursor to two pigments, dark brown and yellow. In the black mice there were only two active genes, one for the precursor and one for an enzyme that produced a black pigment.

Following Cuénot, another geneticist, Sewall Wright (Fig. 3–1), carried out extensive studies on coat color mutants of guinea pigs. In 1917 he published a paper entitled, "Color Inheritance in Mammals" in which he proposed a scheme for the genetic control of pigment formation that, like Cuénot's scheme, involved genes for two enzymes. Wright was a versatile geneticist who greatly influenced the development of genetics during the twentieth century. He not only started to investigate the biochemical basis of gene action, but he also was a pioneer in the development of the field of population genetics.

A very direct demonstration of a gene controlling the production of an enzyme occurred at the same time as Cuénot's studies on mice. The work was not that of a geneticist but of a physician. He became interested in certain rare metabolic aberrations that he encountered in his medical practice.

The physician's name was Archibald Garrod. He was born in 1858, the son of Alfred Garrod, a distinguished clinician and a pioneer in the application of chemistry to medicine. A major contribution of the elder Garrod was the demonstration of high levels of uric acid in patients with gout. The younger Garrod inherited from his father his interest in both medicine and chemistry. During the early years of his medical practice he became interested in the chemistry and clinical significance of urinary pigments. In 1897 he came across a patient with alkaptonuria, characterized by blackening of urine on exposure to air. The study of this condition was to occupy him for years to come.

The black pigment in the urine was shown to be an oxidation product of homogentisic acid, a derivative of the aromatic amino acids tyrosine and phenylalanine, normal protein components. Since alkaptonuria had been found to be a lifelong condition starting in early infancy, Garrod concluded that the abnormality was likely to be hereditary. The conclusion was strengthened by his finding that healthy and apparently normal parents of alkaptonuria patients were frequently first cousins.

The discovery of frequent parental consanguinity giving rise to alkaptonuria occurred in 1901, 1 year after the rediscovery of Mendel's work. It came to Bateson's attention who quickly appreciated the significance and importance of Garrod's discovery. He pointed out to Garrod that the familial distribution of alkaptonuria that he had noted was what would be expected if the abnormality was determined by a recessive (as opposed to dominant) Mendelian factor. In 1902, Garrod published the first substantial account of Mendelian inheritance in man.

In subsequent years Garrod carried out detailed studies on the biochemical disturbance in alkaptonuria. He was convinced that homogentisic acid was an intermediary in the normal conversion process of the aromatic amino acids to carbon dioxide and water. In alkaptonurics, the conversion was blocked after

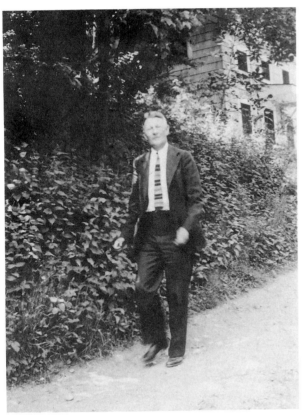

FIGURE 3–1. Sewall Wright, a great pioneer in the fields of Physiological Genetics and Population Genetics, during a visit in Cold Spring Harbor in 1941. [Courtesy of Cold Spring Harbor Laboratory Archives.]

homogentisic acid and therefore this compound accumulated in the urine. In order to analyze the chemical pathway of conversion of aromatic amino acids, he fed alkaptonuric patients aromatic compounds that he thought might be normal precursors of homogentisic acid and tested the patients for increased excretion of homogentisic acid. This method for studying a metabolic pathway by looking for accumulation of intermediates in mutants was used in experiments carried out 40 years later to study biosynthetic pathways in microorganisms.

Garrod also began to study other inherited defects of metabolism that he suspected to be due to a block in a pathway. He reported his studies in 1908 in a series of lectures, later published under the title of, *Inborn Errors of Metabolism.* He proposed a general theory that explained not only the defect in alkaptonuria but also other disorders as well. In essence he suggested that in each condition there was a block at a specific point in the course of normal metabolism and that this was due to the inherited deficiency of a specific enzyme. It was an early form of the one gene–one enzyme hypothesis which 40 years later, following the discoveries of Beadle and Tatum on *Neurospora*, was to play a central role in the development of research on gene action.

Garrod, like Mendel, was ahead of his time and the significance of his work for genetics (although not for biochemistry and medicine) was not appreciated until 40 years later. Unlike Mendel, Garrod was not a geneticist and he did not set out to study genes and their actions. In the end he did however, point out the significance of his experiments for gene action. Why was this not appreciated by geneticists?

Beadle, in a lecture in 1950, gives an explanation which, like other statements of his, is simple and probably correct. In commenting on the neglect of Garrod's work, he stated: "I have often wondered why this was so. I suppose most geneticists were not yet inclined to think of hereditary traits in chemical terms. Certainly biochemists . . . were not keenly aware of the intimate way in which genes direct the reactions of living systems that were the subject of their science."

During two decades following Garrod's work, geneticists concentrated their efforts on elucidating the chromosomal mechanism of gene transmission. Their research, although limited to a defined area, was very productive and brought many new phenomena to light. Some branched out into the related area of embryology. Most geneticists had been zoologists or botanists before they entered the new science of genetics and, as we have seen in the case of Morgan, they had a deep interest in development. In fact, Morgan, while limiting his research to chromosome mechanics, wrote five books about embryology between 1915 and 1935. The subject was always on his mind.

Geneticists concerned with embryology were bound to think about the actions of genes during development. Many genetic aberrations were known that affected different stages of development. Richard Goldschmidt, a zoologist, who had become Second Director of the Kaiser Wilhelm Institut für Biologie in Berlin, was investigating such genetic defects in the development of insects, particularly the gypsy moth *Lymantria*. He found that he could produce the same kinds of defects as mutations do by changing the environmental conditions, especially temperature. He called these changed animals phenocopies. He found that exposure to an altered temperature was effective only at a certain susceptible stage of development.

In thinking about the gene action problem, Goldschmidt concluded that it was not enough for a gene to make a specific enzyme, but it was also important when and where during development the gene produced the enzyme. The gene, therefore, had to be more than a template for making an enzyme or, as some people thought, the enzyme itself. It had to be able to regulate the amount of enzyme produced under different conditions. Goldschmidt, therefore, considered the gene to be a complex entity that could regulate its own activity in response to changes in its environment. This notion was shared by other contemporary geneticists. Because of the often manifold effects of genes (called pleiotropic effects) it seemed to them that genes had to be complex units. It was the prevalence of this notion that prevented them from looking for a straightforward relationship between genes and enzymes as Garrod had visualized.

What Goldschmidt did not consider, and what did not become apparent until 30 years later, was the possibility that there were special regulatory proteins, produced by regulatory genes, whose function it is to control the activity of the other genes that make enzymes. As we mentioned before, at the time of Goldschmidt's experiments between 1910 and 1925 it was not yet known that enzymes were proteins. There was no reason to expand at that time the one gene–one enzyme hypothesis to a one gene–one protein hypothesis, as was done later. (In fact, the first clear demonstration of the one gene–one enzyme hypothesis was in 1949 with human hemoglobin, which is not an enzyme.) As it often happens in biological research, the lack of basic biochemical knowledge can lead to unnecessarily complicated hypotheses. This statement corroborates the above quoted remarks of Beadle.

In the 1930s, studies on gene action shifted toward a more direct approach: to investigate genes and their products. Much of this shift was due to the influence of J.B.S. Haldane. He was a versatile scientist with a solid grounding in both biochemistry and genetics. He received his earliest training as a young boy from his father, J.S. Haldane, who was a distinguished mammalian physiologist in Cambridge, England. As a student he worked in the laboratory of the biochemist Frederick Gowland Hopkins in Cambridge and acquired a solid background in biochemistry. At the same time he was also involved in genetic studies. His main interest was in the interpretation of gene action in terms of biochemical reactions. As he stated in 1942 in his book *New Paths in Genetics* ". . . for if I gained nothing else from ten years' work under so great a biochemist as Hopkins, I gained the conviction that biochemical explanations are more fundamental than morphological [explanations]."

To study gene action, Haldane initiated a research program dealing with the genetics of flower pigments. His colleagues carried out extensive studies in this field and much valuable information was obtained on the biosynthesis of these pigments and the effects of mutations affecting single reaction steps. However, the studies did not contribute much to the elucidation of the gene action problem, presumably because the biochemical conversions involved in pigment formation were too intricate to obtain a clear picture of the action of the genes involved in them.

Of greater importance were Haldane's theoretical contributions to the gene action problem. Already in 1920 he had suggested in a publication that genes produce definite quantities of specific enzymes, with different alleles of a gene producing different amounts of the enzyme. This is similar to the ideas proposed by Wright in 1917 in connection with the genetic control of pigment formation (see page 24). Later Haldane changed his view and proposed that different alleles of a gene produce qualitatively different forms of the enzyme. This was based on the finding that different alleles of a gene for human blood groups determine the production of qualitatively different blood group antigens. This notion of Haldane, as well as other ideas that he proposed, played an important role in the planning of experimental studies on gene action.

The experiments that finally opened the road to the one gene–one enzyme hypothesis originated in studies with insects. The work was initiated by Ernst Caspari in Alfred Kühn's laboratory in Göttingen and by George Beadle and Boris Ephrussi in T.H. Morgan's laboratory at the California Institute of Technology (Caltech) in Pasadena. Morgan and his group had moved there from New York in 1928. The experimental animal in Kühn's laboratory was the meal moth *Ephestia,* in Morgan's laboratory, *Drosophila.*

A favorite trait for genetic studies of *Drosophila* was eye color. From 1910 on, many mutants with altered eye color were isolated and the mutated genes were mapped. As mentioned before, the vermilion mutant, isolated by Bridges, had bright red eyes, in contrast to the darker and dull red eyes of normal flies. It was shown later that in normal flies there were two eye pigments, the red pigment and the brown pigment. Vermilion thus lacked the brown pigment. This lack resulted in the bright red color.

In 1920, Sturtevant studied flies that were mosaics for sex, which was the result of loss of one of the X chromosomes during development of female flies. In these flies, part of the body was male, the other part was female. The vermilion gene is located on the X-chromosome. Sturtevant's flies were heterozygous for vermilion: one of the X chromosomes carried a normal (v^+) vermilion gene and gave rise to eyes with both the brown pigment and the red pigment; the other X chromosome carried a mutant (v) gene and gave rise to eyes with red pigment only. In some mosaic flies, one eye was composed of female cells and had a dark red color due to the presence of both pigments. The other eye was composed of male cells and had the bright red vermilion color due to red pigment only. However, Sturtevant noticed that there were dark red patches with both pigments in the vermilion eyes. He interpreted these findings to mean that in female cells carrying the normal vermilion gene (v^+) a precursor was produced that diffused into the male vermilion eye tissue where it was converted to the brown pigment, in some of the cells.

In Kühn's laboratory an eye color mutant of *Ephestia* had been found that was similar to the vermilion mutant of *Drosophila.* Normally *Ephestia* has black eyes (a^+), the mutant had red eyes (a). The mutation in *Ephestia* affected not only the color of the eyes, but also the color of the testicles and the skin. In the early 1930s, Caspari, a doctoral student, was studying the red eye mutant in *Ephestia*. He had read Sturtevant's 1920 paper about vermilion mosaics and he conceived the idea of testing for a diffusible precursor by using a surgical transplantation technique. To do this, he transplanted mutant testicles (a) into normal caterpillars (a⁺). He observed that the mutant testicles became colored when implanted into normal caterpillars. Thus, as in Sturtevant's mosaics, surrounding tissues with the normal gene produced a diffusible substance that resulted in restoring the normal phenotype in the mutant tissues.

At this point in 1934, Caspari could no longer continue his work. Being Jewish he was dismissed by the Nazis from his position as an assistant to Kühn. He went to the United States, where he became professor at the University of Rochester.

In 1934, Beadle and Ephrussi began to carry out transplantation experiments with *Drosophila* that were similar to Caspari's experiments with *Ephestia*. In the course of these experiments, when they were testing for complementation between mutants to form pigment, they discovered an ingenious method for determining the order of precursors in the pathway of pigment synthesis.

Ephrussi and Beadle came from very different backgrounds. Ephrussi was born in Russia and received his training in France. He studied first the development of sea urchin eggs, than became interested in mammalian systems. He worked in Fauré-Fremiet's tissue culture laboratory at the Rothschild Institute in Paris where he received his PhD in 1932. He then switched to the genetics of development, using a mouse strain that carried a lethal gene. In 1934 he received a fellowship to work with L.C. Dunn at Columbia, who was a leading expert on the genetics and embryology of mice. Somehow he was deflected and he ended up at Caltech in Morgan's group, which had become the New Mecca of genetics.

Beadle grew up on a farm near Wahoo, Nebraska and, like Mendel, as a boy learned the skills of farming from his father. He did his undergraduate work at the University of Nebraska College of Agriculture and from there, at the behest of an inspiring teacher, went to Cornell to do his graduate studies with R.A Emerson on maize genetics. After receiving his PhD in 1931 he went to Morgan's laboratory as a postdoctoral fellow to gain some experience in the chromosomal mechanics of *Drosophila*.

In 1934, news of the German transplantation work reached Caltech and the two young investigators decided to work together on similar experiments with *Drosophila*. Because of Sturtevant's results with mosaics, they chose the vermilion mutant for their first attempts. For their transplantations, they went to Ephrussi's laboratory in Paris because it was better equipped for this delicate work than the laboratory at Caltech.

The development of *Drosophila* proceeds from three larval stages to a pupa to an adult fly. There are small structures called imaginal discs in the larva that give rise to the organs of the adult fly. Thus, there are eye imaginal discs that give rise to the eyes. These eye discs had to be isolated from a larva and transplanted into the abdomen of another larva without killing it. This was a very delicate operation that had to be carried out under a dissecting microscope. It took several months before Ephrussi and Beadle mastered this technique. They finally demonstrated that transplanting eye discs from a vermilion larva into normal larvae gave rise to an implanted eye disc in the abdomen of the adult fly with normal eye color, like that of the host, as expected from Sturtevant's results.

Subsequently Ephrussi and Beadle carried out reciprocal transplantation experiments with pairs of different mutants all of which had eyes like the vermilion mutant and which presumably had a block somewhere in the synthesis of the brown pigment (Fig. 3–2). They put a mutant eye disc into a host with a different mutation to see if the host could restore normal pigment formation in the implanted eye. When testing the vermilion mutant and another mutant called cinnabar they obtained a surprising result. When they used a cinnabar host and a vermilion implanted eye disc, they found complementation between the mutants, that is, the normal eye color was restored in the implanted eye. When they used a vermilion host and a cinnabar implanted disc, there was no complementation. The implanted eye retained the mutant eye color. In thinking about these results it occurred to them that they could be explained by assuming that the genetic blocks in the two mutants are in consecutive steps in the pathway of pigment formation, as shown in Figure 3–3. Step 1 is controlled by the normal vermilion gene and is defective in the vermilion mutant. Step 2 is controlled by the normal cinnabar gene and is defective in a cinnabar mutant. Thus, the cinnabar mutant host can make precursor 1, which can be used by the vermilion implant (unable to make precursor 1), to make pigment. However, the vermilion host cannot make the precursors 1 and 2 and therefore cannot restore pigment formation in the cinnabar mutant implant. Later, as we shall see, this explanation was verified by direct chemical experiments. Since it seemed most likely that each reaction step is controlled by a specific enzyme (see Fig. 3–3), the results support the one gene–one enzyme hypothesis. The same complementation method was of great usefulness in later studies on biosynthetic pathways of *Neurospora* and of *E. coli*.

The work of Ephrussi and Beadle was widely recognized as a new approach to basic problems in the biochemistry of gene action. Their very productive collaboration lasted until 1937. At that point they assumed independent senior positions, Ephrussi in Paris, Beadle at Stanford University in Palo Alto. For Beadle, the work on *Drosophila* eye pigments continued to be his main research endeavor. Ephrussi also did some more work with eye pigments, but this was not his major research.

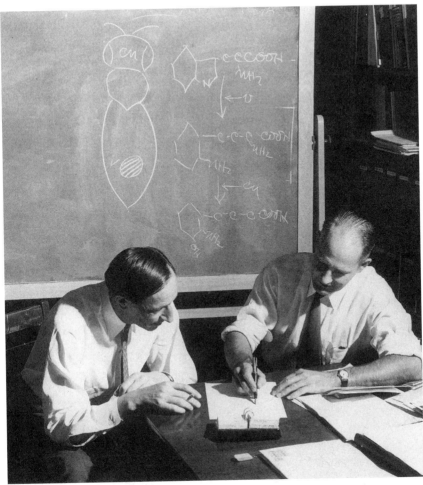

FIGURE 3–2. Boris Ephrussi and George Beadle designing a transplantation experiment to study the steps of brown pigment formation in the 1930s. [Courtesy of California Institute of Technology Archives.]

After 1937 the investigations shifted toward working out the chemical constitution of the pigment precursors, the v^+ and cn^+ substances in *Drosophila* and the a^+ substance in *Ephestia*. For this purpose bioassay methods were developed to demonstrate the presence of these substances in insects. In the course of these studies it was found that the v^+ and a^+ substances could substitute for each other in these assays, suggesting that they were very similar or identical.

Kühn's group in Berlin was joined in 1936 by the eminent organic chemist Adolf Butenandt who set out to determine the chemical nature of the a^+ substance. At about the same time the microbial biochemist Edward Tatum joined

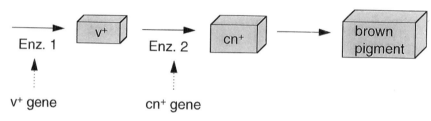

FIGURE 3–3. Scheme for the biosynthesis of the brown pigment, based on the results of the reciprocal transplantation experiment. The cinnabar (cn) mutant host, unable to make enzyme 2, accumulates the vermilion (v⁺) substance, that can "feed" the vermilion (v) mutant implant to make brown pigment. However, the vermilion mutant host, blocked in enzyme 1, cannot make the v⁺ substance and, consequently, the cn⁺ substance; therefore, it cannot "feed" the cinnabar mutant implant, that lacks enzyme 2, to make pigment.

Beadle at Stanford to elucidate the chemistry of the v⁺ and cn⁺ substances. The task of achieving the chemical analysis of these substances turned into a race between the two laboratories. Tatum isolated a substance from a bacterial culture that he knew to be derived from the amino acid tryptophan and that he thought was the v⁺ substance. In the meantime Butenandt identified the v⁺ substance as kynurenine, a derivative of tryptophan. Later the cn⁺ substance was shown to be 3-hydroxykynurenine and to be formed from kynurenine.

After 3 years at Stanford Beadle became discouraged with the slow progress of the eye pigment work. All that he and Tatum had been able to do was to isolate a precursor of the pigment. It had taken thousands of larvae to get enough material for chemical identification. Just as they were ready to carry out the analysis, the chemical structure of the precursor was published by the German group. Beadle felt the necessity of having a better experimental organism for studying the relationship between genes and enzymes and he found it in the breadmold *Neurospora*. Beadle's switch to *Neurospora* was a crucial event. It opened up the field of biochemical genetics, later called molecular genetics. This is the subject of Chapter 4. Before the switch, as a swan song to the Classical Period, he joined Sturtevant in writing a superlative textbook, *An Introduction to Genetics*, which was published in 1939.

4

The *Neurospora* Era

==

THE decision to switch from *Drosophila* to *Neurospora* was made by Beadle while he was listening to Tatum giving a lecture in a course he had organized on comparative biochemistry. With a strong background in the nutrition and biochemistry of bacteria, Tatum was well prepared for this task. His education and doctoral research had convinced him of the validity of the Unity of Biochemistry, the evolutionary conservation of biochemical processes among all living organisms. His theme was that the basic building blocks of life—amino acids, sugars, lipids, growth factors—participated in fundamentally similar chemical pathways among all forms of life. Hence the most fruitful way to study a problem in animal metabolism might be to begin with a microbe that may well prove more convenient for experimental manipulation.

Beadle was sitting in on all of Tatum's lectures. In this particular one, Tatum described the nutrition of yeasts and fungi, some of which exhibited well-defined blocks in vitamin biosynthesis. It was there that Beadle conceived the seminal idea that would alter the future course of genetics. He realized that microbial species could differ in their nutritional requirements, although they shared the same biochemistry. If that were the case, and if these differences were genetic in origin, it should be possible to induce gene mutations that would produce new nutritional requirements in the test organism. If successful, such an approach would reveal genes governing known biochemical reactions immediately, rather than genes for unknown substances, such as the v^+ substance, that required years to identify. As he stated in his autobiographical memoir: "It suddenly occurred to me that it ought to be possible to reverse the procedure we had been following and instead of attempting to work out the chemistry of *known genetic* differences we should be able to select mutants in which *known chemical* reactions were blocked. *Neurospora* was an obvious organism to try this approach."

Neurospora was first described in France in the 1840s. In the warm, humid summer of 1842, bread from the bakeries in Paris was spoiled by massive growth of the orange mold. Subsequently it was studied by a number of microbiologists, who showed that the orange pigment was induced by light. Later, at the beginning of the twentieth century, it was investigated by the Dutch plant physiologist F.A. Went in Indonesia. There it was used, together with peanut meal, in the preparation of a Javanese delicacy, called oncham. It was also conspicuous as the first organism to grow in areas scorched by volcanic eruptions. Went studied the production of secreted enzymes that broke down nutrients such as carbohydrates and proteins.

At the time of Went's studies *Neurospora* was thought to reproduce only asexually, but in the mid-1920s, the botanist B.O. Dodge discovered a sexual phase of reproduction. Dodge had an unusual career. Like Beadle he had grown up on a farm. He worked for years as a school teacher and completed his bachelor's degree only at age 39. He published his first paper at the age of 40 and was already past 50 when he began to work with *Neurospora*, something that became his life's mission. In the next 30 years, he published nearly 50 papers on the genetics, cytology, and life cycle of *Neurospora*. Most of these studies were carried out at the New York Botanical Garden.

Dodge's discovery of the sexual phase made it possible to study genetic recombination and the mapping of genes. He found that there were two mating types (different sexes) whose union resulted in the production of offspring. In the case of *Neurospora*, the nuclei in the vegetatively growing cells contain one set of chromosomes—they are haploid. After union of the parents, the parental nuclei combine to form diploid nuclei. Recombination occurs during a reduction division (meiosis), the recombinant nuclei segregate from each other, and each nucleus becomes incorporated into a spore, called an ascospore. After germination, an ascospore gives rise to vegetatively growing, haploid progeny. Thus, *Neurospora*, like *Drosophila*, has a sexual cycle, but unlike *Drosophila*, the genetic constitution of the mature organism is haploid, whereas in *Drosophila* it is diploid. For genetic studies, *Neurospora* is of advantage, because one can see the genetic constitution of the offspring immediately. It is not obscured, as it is in *Drosophila*, by the presence of a second, dominant form of the gene.

Dodge found that in order to germinate, the ascospores had to be heated. In fact, he had discovered this requirement previously with another mold, when he left a suspension of ascospores in a sterilizing oven that he thought had been turned off. It was presumably the heat activation of spores that was responsible for the early outgrowth of *Neurospora* in French bakeries and after volcanic eruptions.

As Dodge went on with his studies, he became more and more enthusiastic about the advantages of *Neurospora* for genetic studies. He tried to convince Morgan of this and he persuaded him to take some *Neurospora* stocks with him when he moved to his new laboratory at Caltech in 1928. There Morgan maintained the stocks by periodic transfer to fresh medium. At one time while he was doing this, he was visited by a young plant pathologist, Carl Lindegren, who wanted to do graduate work under his guidance. Morgan saw his opportunity and suggested to Lindegren to work on the genetics of *Neurospora*. The latter accepted Morgan's proposal and subsequently carried out extensive genetic studies with various mutants of *Neurospora*.

In 1941, Beadle was familiar with the work that had been carried out with *Neurospora*. He had heard about it on two occasions. In 1928, Dodge had given a seminar at Cornell that Beadle, then a graduate student, attended. He and Barbara McClintock made some useful suggestions to Dodge after his seminar. In 1931, he joined Morgan's group at Caltech and there he met Lindegren who told him about his work. In 1941, he realized that *Neurospora*, being haploid, was more suitable for genetic analysis than *Drosophila* and that for biochemical studies, it was far superior. It could easily be grown in large quantities, making it feasible to isolate cellular constituents for chemical analysis. Its growth was undifferentiated and one did not have to worry about changes that occur during different stages of development. Finally, it could be maintained in pure culture in chemically defined medium and this made it possible to study nutritional requirements as a result of mutation. For *Drosophila* such studies were not possible because there was no chemically defined medium available.

After Tatum's fateful lecture Beadle acted immediately on his insight and wrote to Dodge asking for *Neurospora* stock strains. After their arrival he and Tatum began treatment with X-rays to obtain mutants. They had determined the composition of a simple minimal culture medium consisting of inorganic salts, sucrose, and the vitamin biotin. To look for mutants that could *not* grow in this medium, they first grew the X-rayed spores individually in a rich yeast extract medium that contained many amino acids, vitamins, and other metabolites. On subsequent testing in minimal medium, any that did not grow were considered potential mutants. They were then tested with single growth factors. Among 2000 single spore cultures tested they found three mutants. Each of them required one vitamin for growth, the first vitamin B6 (pyridoxine), the second vitamin B1 (thiamin), the third para-aminobenzoic acid. Five months after receiving the cultures Beadle and Tatum reported their epoch-making results in a paper entitled, "Genetic Control of Biochemical Reactions in *Neurospora.*" The article caused an immediate and widespread stir in the biological community.

In 1941, prior to the publication of the paper, Beadle gave a seminar at Caltech at which he described his findings. Norman Horowitz, then a research fellow at Caltech, described the impact of this seminar as follows: "The talk lasted only half an hour, and when it was suddenly over, the room was silent. The silence was a form of tribute. The audience was thinking; nobody with such a discovery could stop talking about it after just 30 minutes—there must be more. Superimposed on this thought was the realization that something historic had happened. Each one of us, I suspect, was mentally surveying, as best he could, the consequences of the revolution that had just taken place. Finally, when it became clear that Beadle had actually finished speaking, Professor Went— whose father had carried out the first nutritional studies on *Neurospora* in Java at the turn of the century—got to his feet and, with characteristic enthusiasm addressed the graduate students in the room. "This lecture proves," said Went, "that biology is not a finished subject—there are still great discoveries to be made!"

Beadle and Tatum assembled a small group of young investigators that worked together with great enthusiasm and intensity during the next few years on the isolation and biochemical characterization of nutritionally deficient mutants. They included Norman Horowitz, David Bonner, H.K. Mitchell, Mary Houlahan, and two graduate students, A.H Doerman and Adrian Srb. Between 1941 and 1945 this group identified hundreds of mutants, each having a growth requirement for a single vitamin (eight different vitamins), amino acid (eleven different amino acids) and nucleic acid base (four different ones) (Figs. 4–1, 4–2). Studies of these mutants enabled them to work out several unknown steps in basic biochemical pathways and to verify others that had been demonstrated in other organisms. The spirit of this group was comparable to that of the brilliant young investigators assembled around Morgan. As Horowitz describes it: "Now biochemical genetics was a real science, and it was all new. Incredibly, we privileged few had it all to ourselves. Every day brought unexpected new results, new mutants, new phenomena. It was a time when one went to work in the morning wondering what new excitement the day would bring."

A remarkable feature of their studies was that in most mutants a single biochemical reaction was absent. There was apparently a one-to-one relationship between genes and biochemical reaction steps. In turn, this suggested a one-to-one relationship between genes and the enzymes controlling the reaction steps. In 1945 Beadle proposed that the biochemical action of genes could be explained by assuming that genes are responsible for enzyme specificity, the relationship being that "a given enzyme will usually have its final specificity set

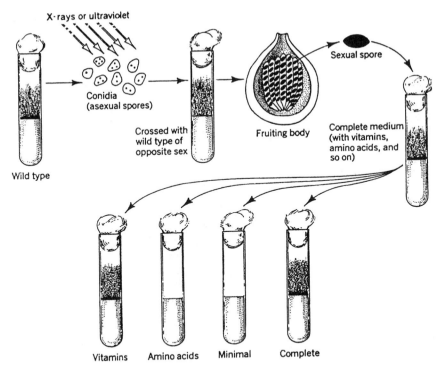

FIGURE 4–1. Outline of the procedure for producing, detecting, and classifying biochemical mutants in *Neurospora*. The illustration indicates that the mutant tested here is deficient in the synthesis of a vitamin. The particular vitamin required for growth could be determined by inoculating the mutant strain into culture tubes containing individual vitamins.

by one and only one gene." This statement became known as the one gene–one enzyme hypothesis of gene action. It is Beadle's major legacy to molecular genetics.

In his Harvey Lecture in 1945, Beadle made the following profound comment about the then current relationship between genetics and biochemistry. "It is perhaps unnecessary to state the obvious conclusion that if one is to understand the metabolism of an organism in the most complete way possible, genes must be taken into account. Too often in the past these units have been regarded as the exclusive property of the geneticist. The biochemist cannot understand what goes on chemically in the organism without considering genes any more than a geneticist can fully appreciate the gene without taking into account what it is and what it does. It is a most unfortunate consequence of human limitations and the inflexible organization of our institutions of higher

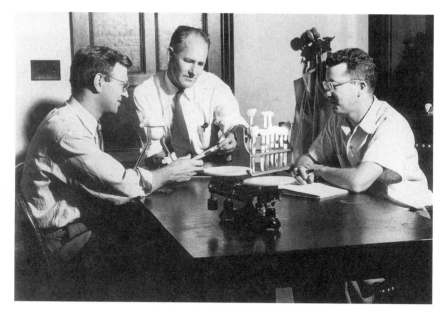

FIGURE 4–2. George Beadle (center) and Norman Horowitz (right) discussing *Neurospora* cultures with a postdoctoral student in the 1940s. The person to the left is unidentified. [Courtesy of California Institute of Technology Archives.]

learning that investigators tend to be forced into laboratories with such labels as biochemistry or genetics. The gene does not recognize the distinction—we should at least minimize it." This was the clarion call to unite geneticists and biochemists for the new age of molecular genetics.

In 1944, Barbara McClintock visited Stanford at Beadle's invitation. Her long experience with maize enabled her to show convincingly that the chromosomes of *Neurospora* and their behavior in the ascus were the same as in higher organisms. She outlined the details of meiosis and described the seven chromosomes. At the end of her 2-month stay there was no longer any question: it was clear that fungal chromosome cytology, like fungal genetics, is basically similar to that of plants and animals.

In 1945 the team of Beadle and Tatum dissolved when Tatum left Stanford for Yale University. In the following year Beadle returned to Caltech—this time to succeed Morgan as chairman of the Division of Biology. He took most of the members of his group with him. They continued their *Neurospora* studies, with most of their efforts being concentrated on working out biochemical pathways. There was rich harvest waiting for them.

In 1946 I came to Caltech as a postdoctoral fellow to learn about *Neurospora*. I had done the research for my PhD thesis at Columbia University on the biochemical genetics of one of the eye pigments of *Drosophila*. After completing my PhD studies I wanted to switch to *Neurospora* and applied for a fellowship at Caltech. As a footnote, the way I was notified illustrates the informal atmosphere of those days. My advisor, T. Dobzhansky, called me into his office one morning and handed me a little slip of paper that said; "Maas accepted, Sturtevant."

I went to Caltech with great expectations. However, in 1946 the initial excitement of the *Neurospora* work had subsided and people had settled down to more or less routine projects dealing with the use of mutants to work out biochemical pathways. The heyday of the *Neurospora* era was over.

My main interest was in finding out more about the ways in which genes controlled the production of enzymes. This problem was being investigated mainly by H.K. Mitchell. In 1948 Mitchell and Lein described the absence of enzyme activity of one of the enzymes of tryptophan biosynthesis in a tryptophan-requiring mutant. In the following year, R. Wagner and B. Guirard at the University of Texas in Austin described a mutant unable to synthesize the vitamin pantothenic acid. Whole cells of the mutant lacked enzyme activity, as expected. Curiously, extracts prepared from the mutant had enzyme activity, which showed that the enzyme, though inactive in intact cells was not eliminated by the mutation. Neither Mitchell and Lein nor Wagner and Guirard could determine the nature of the change in the enzyme protein that resulted in its inactivity. The question of how the gene controls the nature of the corresponding enzyme protein remained unanswered.

I did not see much of Beadle because he was preoccupied with his administrative duties. He did make rounds to the laboratories of the postdocs, but after sticking in his head and asking, "How is it going?" he usually withdrew before one had a chance to engage him in a discussion. A few times I witnessed his simple and direct manner. For example, one morning I arrived early and, passing his office, I saw him vigorously sweeping the floor. I stopped, and noticing my astonished face, he said: "It doesn't matter what you do, as long as you do it well." Another time, as I was walking next to him along the spacious corridor of the floor that housed the *Neurospora* laboratories, he said to me: "At Stanford we worked in a basement under crowded conditions and we produced great work. Now that we have all the space and facilities one could hope for, we will probably never do a damn thing."

Beadle continued to serve as chairman of the Biology Division until 1961. At that time, he accepted an appointment as President of the University of Chicago. There he became even further removed from doing research. However, after his retirement in 1968, he returned to an old interest of his graduate student days, the evolutionary origin of maize, and he spent most of his time and effort in demonstrating that maize originated from a plant called teosinte that grows in Mexico and Guatemala. This was a fitting end to his career.

During my stay at Caltech I often discussed my ideas about gene–enzyme relationships with Norman Horowitz who had become the scientific heir apparent to Beadle. Norm, to his friends, had a sharp and wide-ranging mind, masked by a relaxed and easy-going manner. He had a deep interest in the evolution of biochemical pathways and in the origin of life. In later years, he designed a device for detecting living matter that was mounted on the Viking spaceship that landed on Mars. He sent me a photo of the spaceship on the surface of Mars, with the comment that, "there is no life on Mars." Not quite as famous as Beadle and Tatum at the time of my stay at Caltech, he was already being recognized as the chief advocate of the one gene—one enzyme hypothesis.

One time when I talked to Norm about the experimental problems involved in elucidating gene enzyme relationships, he made a remark that left a deep impression and that was also prophetic: "It is difficult to solve a problem in biology by frontal attack," he said. "You always have to wait until Nature turns her back." As we see in Chapter 6 dealing with *E. coli,* I found a mutant serendipitously that made it possible to see how a gene controls the formation of an enzyme.

5

Escherichia coli
Enters the Field

E SCHERICHIA *coli* (*E. coli*) is a bacterium whose normal habitat is the intestine of man and animals. It is named after Theodor Escherich, a German pediatrician, who first isolated it in 1885 from feces of children whose intestinal function he was studying at the University of Munich. At first, *E. coli*
was considered to be a harmless organism that formed part of the normal intestinal flora. In later years, it was found to be the causative agent of a number of
infectious diseases, including diarrhea, urinary tract infection, and frequently
fatal infections of the blood stream. This paradoxical situation was resolved
when it was found that only certain strains of *E. coli* caused these diseases. In
recent years the characteristics of these strains that are responsible for their
virulence have been an important subject for investigation by medical microbiologists. Outbreaks of diarrheal infections caused by food contaminated with a
virulent strain of *E. coli* have been reported frequently in the daily newspapers.

E. *coli* has properties that make it well suited for biochemical genetics, even
better than *Neurospora*. Like *Neurospora*, it is easily grown in liquid media or
solid media such as agar plates. A liquid culture consists of millions of individual organisms that can be enumerated by inoculating agar plates with serial
dilutions of the culture. Each colony that grows up on an agar plate consists of
a genetically homogeneous clone derived from a single bacterium. Mutants
that arise in a culture can be recognized by plating out dilutions on appropriate

indicator agar media. The cells within the filamentous threads of *Neurospora*, however, contain many nuclei and it is not possible to isolate from them genetically homogenous clones directly. This can best be done from the spores formed after mating with another strain, which is a laborious procedure. *E. coli* grows very rapidly, doubling in less than an hour, giving rise to millions of offspring in a day. Its growth requirements are even simpler than those of *Neurospora*, consisting only of inorganic salts and a sugar as source of carbon and energy. However, with all these advantages, *E. coli* was not used for research in biochemical genetics until the mid-1940s, because it was not known until then that *E. coli* possessed genes and a mating system that was similar to the mating systems in higher forms

Before the 1940s, there was very little contact between bacteriologists and geneticists. Most bacteriologists assumed that the mechanism of inheritance in bacteria was different from that in plants and animals. There were several reasons for this assumption. Bacteria are much smaller than the cells of plants and animals and no nucleus or chromosomes could be discerned in them. It was thought, therefore, that bacteria did not have separate nuclei and chromosomes, but that the organism as a whole acted as the genetic material. Bacterial cultures were found to change rapidly in response to environmental conditions, and these changes were thought to be too rapid to be accounted for on the basis of gene mutations that were known to occur only rarely. What was not appreciated was that bacterial cultures contain millions of individual organisms that can grow rapidly. Rapid changes in a culture can thus be explained on the basis of the presence of a minority of mutants that can outgrow the rest of the population when environmental conditions change. A prevalent idea was that environmental changes could induce changes in the bacteria that were subsequently inherited. Bacteriology was the last stronghold of the Lamarckian view of evolution, which postulated the inheritance of acquired characteristics.

There was one exceptional microbiologist, Martinus Beijerinck, who clearly recognized early the potential of bacteria for genetic studies. He was Professor of Microbiology at the Polytechnic Institute in Delft and was recognized as one of the outstanding microbiologists of his time. In 1900, shortly after De Vries had announced his mutation theory at a meeting of the Royal Academy in Amsterdam, Beijerinck gave a lecture at the same institution, entitled "On Different Forms of Hereditary Variation of Microbes," which he began with these words: "The interesting lecture of Professor Hugo De Vries at the last meeting of the Academy on the origin of new forms in higher plants, induces me to draw attention to some observations regarding the same subject in microbes." He then pointed out that, with microbes, it is easier to start from one individual in the making of cultures, that in these cultures many generations succeed each other quickly, that large numbers of individuals can be surveyed at one time, and that with many microbes the mutability is great, making them especially suitable for the study of heredity.

Beijerinck had been a botanist before becoming a microbiologist and at that time had received a reprint of Mendel's paper. Shortly after he heard De Vries' lecture he sent him the reprint with a note saying: "I know that you are studying hybrids, so perhaps the enclosed reprint of 1865 by a certain Mendel which I happen to possess is still of some interest to you." Presumably it was Beijerinck who called De Vries' attention to Mendel's work.

Over the next two decades Beijerinck was preoccupied with genetics. In 1912, he published a long review entitled "Mutation bei Mikroben" (Mutation Among Microbes), in which he related microbial genetic phenomena in bacteria, fungi and algae to those in higher forms. He emphasized that there is no reason to think that mutants of sexually reproducing organisms should differ from asexually reproducing organisms.

In 1917, Beijerinck published a paper entitled "The Enzyme Theory of Heredity." There he considered the possibility that genes and enzymes could be regarded as identical. He speculated that, if that is the case, new light is thrown on the nature and on the action of genes during development, and also on the occurrence of fluctuating variability and of mutations.

After microbial genetics became established as a discipline in the late 1940s Beijerinck did not receive the general recognition that Garrod had received as the "founder of the one-gene–one-enzyme hypothesis." It seems to me that, Beijerinck, with his prophetic insight into the potentialities of bacteria for genetics deserves to be recognized more widely as a pioneer.

The first clear evidence that *E. coli* possesses genes like those of higher forms was the demonstration in 1943 that genetic changes in *E. coli* are not induced by the environment, but that they occur randomly and with the same low frequency as mutations in higher forms. The key experiment was carried out by Salvador Luria, an Italian physician turned radiobiologist, who had become interested in bacterial viruses, and Max Delbrück, a German physicist, who had also become interested in bacterial viruses. What brought Luria and Delbrück together was the shared idea that bacterial viruses, usually called bacteriophages, because of their small size and simple chemical constitution—they contain only proteins and nucleic acids—could serve as a model system to study the replication and action of genes.

Luria began work on bacteriophage in 1938 in the laboratory of the bacteriologist Geo Rita in Rome, but, being Jewish, he could not get a job in Italy. He went to the Institute of Radium in Paris to continue his studies on the inactivation of bacteriophages by X-rays. Forced to leave France when the Germans entered in 1940, he came to the United States where he continued his work at Columbia University with financial support from the Rockefeller Foundation. Luria met Delbrück, whose papers he had read earlier, at a meeting in

Philadelphia in 1940. They became friends immediately and began a collaboration in Luria's laboratory at Columbia University.

Max Delbrück came from an intellectual family in Prussia. His father was a professor of history a the University of Berlin. His early training was in physics, first in astrophysics and then in theoretical physics. A lecture by the Danish physicist Niels Bohr in 1932 on "Light and Life" aroused his interest in biology. Bohr thought that the study of biology could lead to the discovery of new principles of physics. Shortly after this lecture Delbrück became Lise Meitner's assistant in Otto Hahn's laboratory at the Kaiser Wilhelm Institute for chemistry in Berlin. There he became interested in genetics. Influenced by Muller's discovery of the mutagenic action of X-rays he joined up with the Russian geneticist N.W. Timoféef-Ressovsky and the physicist K.G. Zimmer in a study using the mutagenic effect of ionizing radiation to measure the physical volume of the gene. The three wrote a paper entitled, "On the Nature of Gene Mutations and Gene Structure," which is of fundamental importance in the history of molecular genetics, because it assigned a chemical reality to the gene. Because of the repressive state of Nazi Germany at the time, Delbrück went to Caltech in 1937 with financial support from the Rockefeller Foundation. Previously in Berlin, he had met Warren Weaver, the head of this foundation, who played an important part in promoting the recruitment of chemists and physicists into biology. He selected Caltech because of T.H. Morgan, but he quickly decided that *Drosophila* was too complicated for him and chose to work on the replication of bacteriophage. Together with Emory Ellis he carried out fundamental studies on the growth of bacteriophages that infect *E. coli*. Although Delbrück's Rockefeller Foundation fellowship terminated in 1939, the poilital situation in Germany prevented him from returning there. With further help from the Rockefeller foundation, a position was found for him in the Physics Department of Vanderbilt University, where he remained from 1940 until the end of World War II.

The key experiment that demonstrated the spontaneous occurrence of bacterial mutations was an offshoot of Luria's studies on bacteriophages of *E. coli*. He was studying the multiplication of the bacteriophages (usually called phages) by infecting bacterial cultures with phages. In about 30 minutes after infection, the bacteria lysed and each bacterium released several hundred phages into the medium. However, there were always a few bacteria that did not lyse and survived the infection. They were resistant mutants. Luria began to wonder about the origin of the resistant mutants. Were they induced by exposure to the bacteriophage? Or were they present in the culture before infection and were merely selected out by the bacteriophage?

The answer came in January 1943, just after he had joined the faculty of Indiana University in Bloomington. One evening he was attending a dance at the Bloomington Country Club. During the intermission he was watching a colleague gambling on a slot machine. In his words, "though losing most of the time he occasionally got a return. Not a gambler myself, I was teasing him about his inevitable losses, when he suddenly hit the jackpot. He gave me a dirty look and walked away. Right then I began giving some thought to the actual numerology of slot machines; in so doing, it dawned on me that slot machines and bacterial mutations may have something to teach each other."

What impressed Luria was the uneven return from the slot machine, with jackpots being rare events. He compared these returns with the presumed occurrence of mutations to phage resistance in growing cultures. These are also rare events. If the mutations occurred by chance, prior to phage infection, then in a series of 100 culture tubes, each inoculated with a few bacteria and grown to full density, most mutations would occur at the end of growth when many bacteria were present. However, there was a small chance that mutations would occur early during the growth when few bacteria were present. To score the number of resistant mutants, phages were added to each tube at the end of growth and, after incubation and lysis of the bacteria, the number of surviving bacteria were counted by plating on media where these survivors could grow out into colonies. Since mutations are rare events most tubes would have only a few survivors. However, in tubes where a mutation had occurred early during growth, there would be many survivors, these being the offspring of the cell in which the mutation had occurred. In other words, there would be a few "jackpot" tubes.

However, if the mutations were induced by the phages they would occur only after phage infection, which is done at the end of growth, and the chance for mutations to occur would be the same for all tubes. In other words, there would be *no* "jackpot" tubes. Luria was very excited about this idea and immediately put it to the test. The results were clearly in favor of the spontaneous origin of mutants. Samples taken from many independent bacterial cultures gave him rare "jackpot" tubes, whereas many duplicate samples taken from the same culture did not.

Luria communicated his results to Delbrück at Vanderbilt University. Delbrück replied immediately: "You are right about the difference in fluctuations in resistant bacterial colonies, when the sampling is done from one or from many cultures. I think what this problem needs is a worked out and written down theory, and I have begun doing so."

Thus was born what is usually called the Luria-Delbrück Fluctuation Test (Fig. 5–1). The results of the test showed unequivocally that the genetic changes arise spontaneously during the growth of cultures and in the absence of the bacteriophage. The same results were found with genetic changes that made bacteria resistant to other inhibitory agents such as antibiotics. Suddenly, biologists began to accept the notion that bacteria had genes, similar to those in higher forms of life. At the time this was a radical change in their thinking. The

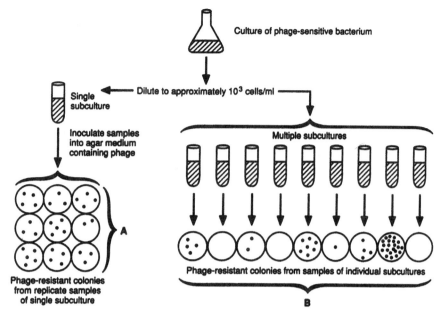

FIGURE 5–1. Schematic presentation of the Luria-Delbrück fluctuation test. Tube number 8 in B (second from right) is a "jackpot" culture, in which a mutation to phage resistance occurred early during the growth of the culture, thus giving rise to many phage-resistant bacteria.

experiment was also a cornerstone in the history of genetics, because it was the first in a series of discoveries that established *E. coli* as the favored experimental material for molecular genetics.

After 1943, Luria and Delbrück continued to study the replication of bacteriophages and began to unravel the genetic constitution of these organisms. In this effort they were joined by A.D. Hershey, a biochemist. The three formed the nucleus of the Phage Group, whose work played a crucial role in the development of molecular genetics. Some years later, in 1969, Luria, Delbrück and Hershey jointly received a Nobel Prize.

During the summer months, starting in 1941, Luria and Delbrück and their coworkers carried out their work at the laboratory of the Carnegie Institution of Washington at Cold Spring Harbor, which is located near Huntington, Long Island. This laboratory has had a long history in genetic research. In spite of its limited facilities, it has spawned a lot of important work. It is also famous for its yearly symposia, most of which deal with genetics. The director at the time, M. Demerec, who carried out research on *Drosophila* genetics, was farsighted enough to see in the early 1940s the future possibilities of microbial genetics. He recognized the fundamental value of the work of Luria and Delbrück and invited them to carry out their studies during the summer at Cold Spring Harbor. Demerec's attitude is illustrated by the following quotation, which he wrote in defense of the reorientation of his research program to microbial genetics:

> You may properly ask what is the purpose of this research, and why we use microorganisms in our investigations. The answer to this is very simple. By using as experimental material these microorganisms, which are easy to handle, biologists and biochemists are trying to unravel two of the most intricate puzzles of all living matter; namely, the mechanism of heredity, and the reproduction of living substances. Since the fundamental laws of nature are general, discoveries made by working with these minute organisms help us to understand the life processes of higher living beings.

The practical utility of Demerec's prophetic statement was soon proven, when, in the summer of 1945, Luria and Delbrück started to teach the Phage Course, which over the years was attended by many prominent microbiologists and biochemists and was instrumental in spreading the importance of bacteriophage for molecular genetics. The course also attracted physicists who after World War II, for one reason or another, had become disillusioned with physics or, like Delbrück, saw new opportunities in the genetics of microbes.

Actually at that time, Delbrück realized that the great expectations that had led him to study bacteriophages were not fulfilled. He has described this situation in a Harvey Lecture in 1946, as follows:

> You might wonder how such naïve outsiders get to know about the existence of bacterial viruses. Quite by accident, I assure you. Let me illustrate by reference to an imaginary theoretical physicist, who knew little about biology in general, and nothing about bacterial viruses in particular, and who accidentally was brought into contact with this field. Let us assume that this imaginary physicist was a student of Niels Bohr, a teacher deeply familiar with the fundamental problems of biology, through tradition, as it were, he being the son of a distinguished physiologist, Christian Bohr.
>
> Suppose now that our imaginary physicist, the student of Niels Bohr, is shown an experiment in which a virus particle enters a bacterial cell and 20 minutes later the bacterial cell is lysed and 100 virus particles are liberated. He will say: "How come, one particle has become 100 particles of the same kind in 20 minutes?" That is very interesting. Let us find out how it happens! How does the particle get in to the bacterium? How does it multiply? Does it multiply like a bacterium, growing and dividing, or does it multiply by an entirely different mechanism? Does it have to be inside the bacterium to do this multiplying, or can we squash the bacterium and have the multiplication go on as before? Is this multiplying a trick of organic chemistry which the organic chemists have not yet discovered? Let us find out. This is so simple a phenomenon that the answers cannot be hard to find. In a few months we will know. All we have to do is to study how conditions will influence the multiplication. We will do a few experiments at different temperatures, in different media, with different viruses, and we will know. Per-

haps we may have to break into the bacteria at intermediate stages between infection and lysis. Anyhow, the experiments only take a few hours each, so the whole problem can not take long to solve.

Perhaps you would like to see this childish young man after eight years, and ask him, just offhand, whether he has solved the riddle of life yet? This will embarrass him, as he has not got anywhere in solving the problem he set out to solve. But being quick to rationalize his failure, this is what he may answer, if he is pressed for an answer: "Well, I made a slight mistake. I could not do it in a few months. Perhaps it will take a few decades, and perhaps it will take the help of a few dozen other people. But listen to what I have found, perhaps you will be interested to join me."

In 1945, as a result of the Luria-Delbrück Experiment and the work of the Phage Group, the existence of genes in bacteria was generally accepted. What was lacking was a mating system that made it possible to carry out genetic analysis.

Such a system was found in 1946 by Joshua Lederberg, working in the laboratory of Tatum at Yale University (Fig. 5–2).

Lederberg grew up in New York City. He was a precocious youngster with a vital interest in science, especially in biology. As a student at Stuyvesant High School, which specializes in science, he found the encouragement and opportunities he needed to pursue his interests. He also read widely on his own on scientific subjects. When he entered Columbia College in 1941, he was well prepared to take full advantage of the opportunities offered in the science curriculum.

A pivotal event for Lederberg was his encounter in 1942 with Francis Ryan, who had done his postdoctoral studies with Tatum and Beadle at Stanford, and was an assistant professor in the Zoology Department. From Ryan he learned about the exciting developments in the biochemical genetics of *Neurospora.* Soon he associated himself with Ryan in the laboratory work on mutants of *Neurospora* and he continued to carry out experiments with this mold throughout his college years.

Lederberg entered Columbia College of Physicians and Surgeons as a medical student in October 1944 but he still maintained his contact with Ryan's laboratory. Toward the end of his first year, in the spring of 1945, he conceived the idea of testing for the occurrence of sexual reproduction in bacteria. Based on the crosses made with nutritionally deficient mutants of *Neurospora,* his protocol was to mix cultures of two such mutants, say A^+B^- and A^-B^+, and plate them on a minimal medium agar, on which neither mutant could grow, but an A^+B^+ recombinant could do so. To be sure that such growth was not due to reverse mutation, for example, A^-B^+ to A^+B^+, he proposed to use cultures of double mutants, such as $A^-B^-C^+D^+$ and $A^+B^+C^-D^-$. With such strains, reversion of two mutations would be required and the chance of that happening would be extremely rare.

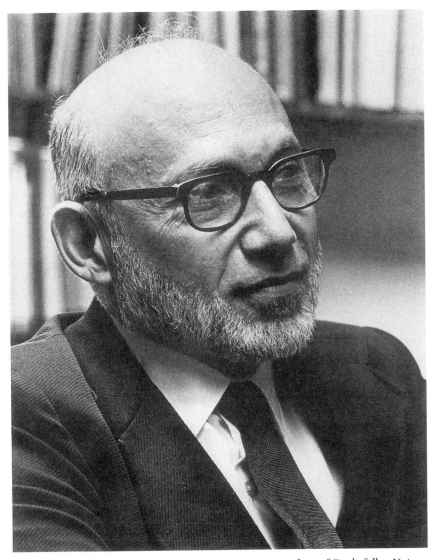

Figure 5–2. Joshua Lederberg during his tenure as President of Rockefeller University. [Courtesy of Joshua Lederberg.]

An opportunity to test his idea about sex in bacteria arose in 1946 in the laboratory of Tatum, who had recently moved to Yale University. In fact, it was Ryan who suggested to him to contact Tatum. The latter started to work with *E. coli* and had isolated double mutants, of the kind that Lederberg was looking for. One of these required the vitamin biotin and the amino acid methionine for growth, whereas the other required the amino acids threonine and proline.

Tatum invited Lederberg to carry out his proposed experiments at Yale, and Lederberg went there in the spring of 1946, on a leave of absence from medical school. Within 6 weeks after his arrival he demonstrated the occurrence of sexual reproduction in bacteria by using Tatum's two double mutant strains.

This epoch-making discovery clinched the use of *E. coli* for genetic studies. Lederberg and Tatum presented their results at the Cold Spring Harbor Symposium on "Genetics of Microorganisms" in the summer of 1946. Their short paper caused a tremendous stir. Later, in 1958, this work gained for Lederberg, who was at the time of his discovery 21 years old, a Nobel Prize with Tatum and Beadle.

Lederberg did not finish medical school. In 1946, he took another leave of absence to complete his work on the mating of *E. coli* strains. During this time, he was offered a position as assistant professor at the University of Wisconsin in Madison, which gave him the opportunity to develop the field of bacterial genetics. This enticement outweighed his desire to finish his medical studies. Before Lederberg left for Madison, Yale University, with the help of Tatum, granted him a PhD degree.

Lederberg and Tatum were lucky in their choice of a strain of *E. coli*, called *E. coli* K12, which Tatum had acquired from the stock culture collection of Stanford's Microbiology Department. It turned out later that only a small fraction of *E. coli* strains, 1 in 20, are fertile in matings. A strain of *E. coli*, called *E. coli* B, which Demerec and Delbrück had insisted upon as a standard strain, is infertile and attempts to obtain sexual reproduction with this strain would have been unfruitful. This situation is similar to Mendel's choice of seven genes, that did not exhibit any linkage in his crosses. They were located either on different chromosomes or, if they were on the same chromosome, they were far enough from each other to assort independently. Since there are only seven chromosomes in peas, the chance of each gene being located in a different chromosome is very small. If two or more genes had been present in the same region of one of the chromosomes, the corresponding traits would not have been segregated independently and this might have prevented Mendel from recognizing the rules of inheritance. It seems that in the case of Lederberg as well as in that of Mendel, chance was on the side of genius.

Although the choice of *E. coli* K12 was serendipitous, it was vital to Lederberg's success that he had followed a course throughout his studies that eventually led him to his crucial experiments. After entering Columbia University, he seemed to know were he was going. He chose Ryan, who was *not* a famous geneticist, as his mentor, because he found what he needed in Ryan's personality and in his work. Ryan, an energetic young man, was impressed with Lederberg's drive and knowledge and supported him warmly in his laboratory work and in planning his career. Lederberg chose microorganisms for his studies, first *Neurospora* and then *E. coli*, because he recognized their potential for genetics. Thus, by following a path independent of the fashions of the day, he put himself in a position where a lucky finding led to a major scientific advance.

At the University of Wisconsin, Lederberg continued to carry out experiments designed to elucidate the mechanism of genetic recombination he and Tatum had discovered in *E. coli* K12. He assumed that the mechanism was similar to genetic recombination in higher forms and he tried to fit the data he obtained in his matings into the scheme used in the analysis of crosses carried out with *Neurospora* and *Drosophila*. He could not fit his results into this scheme without considerable contortions and, as it turned out in the early 1950s, the mechanism of gene transfer and recombination in *E. coli* was quite different from that in higher forms, as is shown in Chapter 10.

For the analysis of his matings Lederberg, together with his wife Esther M. Lederberg, developed an ingenious method, called *replica plating*. In this procedure colonies are picked up from an agar plate by a velvet disc and "printed" from this disc onto other agar plates of different constitutions. This method made it possible to test many colonies simultaneously. Using this method, Lederberg demonstrated directly that mutations to drug resistance arose in the absence of the drug, as Luria and Delbrück postulated in their fluctuation tests.

In 1950, Norton Zinder, a graduate student of Lederberg, made an important discovery that greatly affected the future course of genetics. He found in *Salmonella typhimurium*, a bacterium closely related to *E. coli*, that there was a second method of gene transfer that did not require contact between the bacteria, as was the case for the conjugative transfer discovered by Lederberg and Tatum. Instead, genes were transferred from one strain to another by a bacteriophage. The process was called transduction and the bacteriophages that could carry out this process were called transducing phages. Gene transfer by transduction has since been demonstrated in many organisms, not only in bacteria but also in higher forms including animals and man where transduction is carried out by viruses. It is of great general importance in medicine and in bioengineering. In bacteria, it makes it possible to detect recombination between genes with a very high resolving power and the method has been used extensively in what is called fine structure mapping.

6

Biochemical Genetics
in *Escherichia coli*

I N 1948, Lederberg and Zinder discovered an efficient method for enriching
mutants that are blocked in biosynthetic pathways and therefore require essential metabolites for growth as is the case in *Neurospora*. This method takes
advantage of the property of penicillin to kill bacteria only when they are growing. Thus, when a mixture of normal and mutant bacteria are inoculated into a
medium where only the normal bacteria can grow, addition of penicillin will kill
the normal bacteria and the mutant bacteria survive. This ingenious and powerful method was discovered at the same time independently by Bernard
Davis, a newcomer who became interested in biochemical genetics after previously carrying out research on tuberculosis. As we see in this chapter, it was
mainly in Davis' laboratory that the fruits of the penicillin method were used to
continue with *E. coli* the tradition of biochemical genetics, started in *Neurospora* (Fig. 6–1). This led to the elucidation of the role of genes in enzyme
formation.

Bernard Davis' early training was in biochemistry and general physiology. As
an undergraduate biochemistry major at Harvard he carried out research on
the dissociation curve of hemoglobin. As a student at Harvard Medical School
he worked in the laboratory of E.J. Cohn, a pioneer in protein chemistry. He
was a brilliant student and graduated with the very rare honor of MD summa
cum laude.

After an internship at Johns Hopkins Hospital, Davis decided to enter a career in medical research and in 1942 became a commissioned officer in the U.S. Public Health Service. He was assigned to study biological false-positive tests for syphilis. To prepare himself for this task, he spent 2 years in New York City in the laboratories of the noted immunologist Elvin Kabat. In 1945 the U.S. Public Health Service offered him his own laboratory to work on basic science problems related to tuberculosis. In preparation, he spent 2 years at the Rockefeller Institute in the laboratory of the eminent microbiologist René Dubos. He contracted a mild case of tuberculosis and had to undergo surgery followed by a protracted recovery period. It was during this time of reading and reflection that he decided to do research in biochemical genetics. The deciding factor was the reading of a review by Beadle on the use of biochemical mutants of *Neurospora* as tools for genetic and biochemical studies. As he stated in an autobiographical memoir in 1992, "It seemed to me that such work on universally distributed biosynthetic pathways should be deeply satisfying because it was near the trunk of the evolutionary tree, while attempts to grow bigger and better tubercle bacilli were only twigs."

Davis set up his laboratory called the Tuberculosis Research Laboratory (although during its existence from 1947 to 1954 it hardly ever saw a tubercle bacillus) at Cornell Medical College in New York City. The laboratory was located in a secure corner of the Department of Preventive Medicine, yet it was in a scientifically central position near the Rockefeller Institute. He surrounded himself with a small group of young associates to investigate the bio-

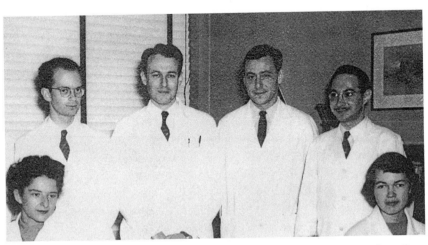

FIGURE 6–1. Bernard Davis and members of his group circa 1950. Standing, from right to left: Henry Vogel, Werner Maas, Bernard Davis, Gordon Allen. Allen later became a human geneticist. Sitting, on the right: Margaret Sanderson, Maas' assistant; on the left: Elizabeth Mingioli, Davis' assistant.

chemical genetics of *E. coli*. Shortly after setting up the laboratory, he conceived of the penicillin enrichment method for the isolation of nutritionally deficient or, as he named them, auxotrophic mutants, and the success of this method put his research into high gear. During the first year he isolated an arsenal of mutants that in its number and variety surpassed the *Neurospora* mutants isolated over a previous 7-year period.

Davis was a microbial physiologist at heart whose aim was to work out cellular mechanisms. These included metabolic reactions and processes associated with it such as the transport of nutrients into the cell. He recognized that mutants could be used as "living dissection needles" to work out metabolic processes. Although he was not a geneticist, he had a deep interest in the physiological functions of genes.

I joined Davis' group in 1948 after my return from Caltech. Davis was looking for a genetically oriented collaborator who would help him exploit the opportunities offered by his plethora of mutants. After a 3-hour stimulating lunch conversation he asked me to become a member of his group and I was happy to accept. This was the beginning of a 10-year long fruitful association, first at Cornell Medical College, and after 1954 at New York University School of Medicine. We complemented each other in our approaches to biology and we worked well together in designing experiments and writing papers.

The major emphasis of the laboratory was on the use of mutants to elucidate biosynthetic pathways. These studies led to the discovery of an entirely new pathway, the synthesis of the three aromatic amino acids tyrosine, phenylalanine, and tryptophan from a common precursor shikimic acid. This compound had originally been isolated from the fruit of the oriental shikimi tree by the chemist H.O.L. Fischer. With the use of mutants, Davis and his associates worked out all the steps leading from shikimic acid to the three aromatic amino acids.

During this period, Davis carried the gospel of the use of *E. coli* for biochemical genetics to Caltech where he taught a summer course in Beadle's department. He also took the phage course at Cold Spring Harbor and became acquainted with Max Delbrück.

The work on biosynthetic pathways constituted the bread-and-butter research of the laboratory. The studies with the *E. coli* mutants also led in directions that were not as clearly defined as biosynthetic pathways but were of great general interest and foreshadowed developments in molecular biology. One of these was the work of Charles Gilvarg and Howard Green, which demonstrated the existence of specific transport systems for individual metabolites. Later they were called *permeases* by Jaques Monod.

A topic in which I had a special interest was the manner in which a gene controlled the production of a specific enzyme. Does it determine the chemical structure of an enzyme, and if so, how? Or does it merely control the rate at which an enzyme is produced?

There is a type of mutant, already described in *Neurospora*, which is favorable material for studying this question. These mutants are so-called temperature-sensitive mutants in which the mutation is expressed only at elevated temperatures. At lower temperatures they behave like normal strains. For example, a mutant was isolated in *Neurospora* that required methionine for growth above 30°C but not below that temperature. Assuming that a gene controls the structure of an enzyme, one would expect that in such a mutant the enzyme is less stable and therefore more rapidly inactivated at elevated temperatures than the corresponding enzyme of the normal strain. In *Neurospora*, no studies on the heat stability of enzymes in temperature-sensitive mutants had been carried out.

By chance I found a temperature-sensitive mutant in *E. coli* in which the enzyme affected by the mutation could be extracted and its activity could be measured in extracts. The enzyme catalyzed the formation of pantothenic acid from two precursors, beta-alanine and pantoic acid. This is the same reaction that was studied by R. Wagner in *Neurospora*, as mentioned previously. I found that in extracts the enzyme extracted from the temperature-sensitive mutant was inactivated at elevated temperatures much more rapidly than the enzyme extracted from the normal strain. This was the first direct demonstration of increased heat lability of a protein as a result of mutation. It showed that this mutation alters the stability rather than the rate of formation of an enzyme protein. From this it was inferred that genes act by determining the structure of enzyme molecules. The 1952 paper by Maas and Davis describing this work was the first evidence that mutations affect the structure of an enzyme not the enzyme-synthesizing apparatus. The following year Horowitz and Fling found a gene in *Neurospora* that determines the thermostability of the enzyme tyrosinase.

The insight gained from the experiments with the temperature-sensitive mutants provided an explanation for a medically important problem. Davis had been isolating mutants that were resistant to the action of various sulfa drugs such as sulfanilamide. These drugs were widely used for the treatment of infections caused by bacteria. Sulfa drugs inhibit the growth of bacteria by interfering with the biosynthesis of folic acid, an essential metabolite. It was known which enzymatic reaction in the formation of folic acid is inhibited by the drugs. In analogy with the temperature-sensitive mutants, Davis postulated that in this case the mutation to resistance resulted in the alteration of the structure of the target enzyme so that it no longer combined with sulfa drugs but could still carry out its normal function in the synthesis of folic acid. Emergence of mutants resistant to growth-inhibiting agents such as antibiotics has to this day remained the most serious limitation in the use of antibiotics. Resistance as a result of an altered enzyme, proposed in the paper by Davis and Maas in 1952, has been shown to be a frequent cause of drug resistance.

In the meantime, Norman Horowitz at Caltech, together with his associate Urs Leupold, had isolated 161 temperature-sensitive mutants of *E. coli*. This was done to answer a criticism of Max Delbrück that challenged the validity of the one gene–one enzyme hypothesis. Delbrück maintained that in the previous method used for mutant isolation, mutants with complex nutritional requirements, and therefore defective in several enzymes, would not be detected. If this criticism were valid, and if mutants with multiple metabolic defects were a significant fraction of the total, then this should be revealed by the analysis of temperature-sensitive mutants, which are selected only for their failure to grow at elevated temperatures on the standard minimal medium. As it turned out, most of the 161 temperature-sensitive mutants could grow at elevated temperatures on the standard complete medium that had been used in previous mutant isolation experiments. They were shown to have single requirements at the elevated temperatures. These results answered Delbrück's objection and were strong support for the one gene–one enzyme hypothesis.

Temperature-sensitive mutants are especially valuable because they make it possible to detect mutant genes whose absence would be lethal. These conditional lethal mutants made it possible to study enzymatic reactions that were not amenable to the available methods of biochemical analysis, such as enzymes controlling the synthesis of DNA. Temperature-sensitive mutants, even if the affected functions are not known, can serve as useful "marker" genes in mapping experiments. Neither Horowitz nor Davis and I were aware of these useful functions of conditional lethal mutants. It took 13 years before this usefulness of such conditional mutants was realized.

At that time, in 1964, R.S. Edgar at Caltech isolated temperature-sensitive mutants of bacteriophage T4 that were affected in various stages of phage development. He put these mutants to good use in studies on phage development and in the construction of a genetic map of phage T4. At about the same time, a colleague of Edgar at Caltech, R.H. Epstein, discovered another kind of conditional lethal mutant in phage T4, which he named *amber* mutants. This name had an unusual origin. One of Epstein's students was named Bernstein and Epstein told him that, if they found the kind of mutant they were looking for, he would name it after his mother. The English translation of Bernstein is amber. Amber mutants could not grow in *E. coli*, unless the strain carried an amber-suppressor mutation in its chromosome that was able to correct the defect produced by the amber mutation in the phage. After the studies of Edgar and Epstein, conditional lethal mutants became favorite tools for the study of vital functions that could not be analyzed by the use of ordinary mutations. The biochemical basis of amber mutations and amber-suppressor mutations was subsequently clarified in studies on the genetic code (see Chapter 11). They were found to cause termination of a growing peptide chain during protein synthesis (see Chapter 9).

In his biographical chapter in 1992, Davis stated: "We [he and I] often discussed ways of generalizing this finding (the altered enzyme in the temperature-sensitive pantothenate mutant), but we failed to formulate clearly the later concept of conditionally lethal mutants. Any scientist can look back and see boats he should not have missed, but this was a large one."

At about the same time as the experiments with *E. coli* mutants were carried out, there was another demonstration of a mutation giving rise to an altered protein. This was not done with *Neurospora* or with *E. coli*, but with man, and the protein was not an enzyme. Linus Pauling and his coworkers at Caltech showed that the hemoglobin produced by people with sickle-cell anemia, an inherited disease, is different in its electric charge from normal hemoglobin. In 1957, it was shown by Vernon Ingram that this difference is caused by the replacement of a particular residue of the amino acid glutamic acid by another amino acid, valine, in the hemoglobin molecule.

The results of the work with temperature-sensitive mutants from Horowitz's laboratory and our laboratory were reported at the 1951 Cold Spring Harbor Symposium on "Genes and Mutations." This was contrary to the general spirit of the symposium, which appeared to cast doubts not only on the one gene–one enzyme hypothesis, but on the existence of genes as separate entities. It was opened by Richard Goldschmidt, who proclaimed that "There was no such thing as a gene, rather that the chromosome was the unit of function and mutations were no more than analogs to stops on the string of a violin." This statement was supported by some mystifying reports that followed. One speaker, J.H. Taylor, stated: "I wish I could say something in behalf of the recently deceased, the gene, but . . ." The only presentations that supported the reality of the one gene–one enzyme hypothesis were the lecture by Horowitz, followed by short presentations by Davis and myself.

This symposium was a last-ditch effort by defenders of an attitude that could not accept the notion that the gene was a basic entity whose chemical constitution could be defined and whose action could be explained in terms of chemical reactions. Biology had to be complicated. Two years later, with the unveiling of the double helix structure of DNA, this attitude began to change. With the known structure of DNA it became possible to envisage how the information contained in the sequence of nucleic acid bases could be transcribed into the sequence of amino acids in protein molecules, just as the association of genes with chromosomes made it possible to envisage Mendel's rules of gene transmission. The credibility of the one gene–one enzyme hypothesis was on its way.

7

The Chemical Nature of Genes

SO far I have described how between 1940 and 1952, studies starting with externally observable characteristics of mutants led to the conclusion that each gene determines the structure of a protein molecule. To study gene action in the reverse direction, starting from chromosomes, it was first necessary to know the chemical nature of genes. This was determined during the same period.

The organism in which the chemical nature of the gene was discovered was a bacterium, *Streptococcus pneumoniae* (commonly known as pneumococcus), a causative agent of pneumonia. The major credit for this discovery goes to three scientist–physicians at the Rockefeller Institute for Medical Research in New York City: Oswald T. Avery, the head of the laboratory, and his two associates, Colin M. MacLeod and Maclyn McCarty.

At the beginning of the twentieth century, prior to the advent of antibiotics, pneumonia was a major cause of death. Most of this devastating disease was caused by pneumococci. Seen under a microscope, these bacteria are little spheres, pointed at one end, and often occurring in pairs. On staining, they are seen to be surrounded by a halo, called a capsule. This structure is important for producing disease. Sometimes, strains are found that do not have a capsule, and they do not cause pneumonia. Strains without a capsule were labeled R (for rough) and strains with a capsule were labeled S (for smooth). This designation is based on the appearance of the colonies when the bacteria are grown on solid agar media. Only S strains produce disease.

Many efforts were made to prevent the growth of pneumococci and, thus, to control the disease. Among these, the use of antisera proved to be effective. It had been found that rabbits or horses, when injected with dead or weakened pneumococci, developed substances in their blood that could protect mice (which are very sensitive to pneumococci) and eventually humans against the disease. These substances were called antibodies and the substances in the bacteria that elicited antibodies were called antigens.

It was found that the capsule was the structure in the S. pneumococci that acted as the major antigen. Antibodies against the capsule were protective against disease. Moreover, it was shown that there were different types of antibodies produced by strains that had antigenically different capsules. For example, type I strains contained a capsule that elicited type I antibodies. These antibodies protect against infection with type I strains, but not against infection with other types. In 1915, there were 4 types known. (Today there are about 80 known types.)

In 1928, Fred Griffith, a medical officer in the Ministry of Health in London, carried out some experiments with pneumococci that revealed a new and very puzzling phenomenon. Griffith was analyzing different antigenic types isolated from patients. One observation that intrigued him was that a single sputum sample from a pneumonia patient could harbor several antigenic types. To explain this he postulated that within the patient one antigenic type could be converted into another type. This led him to carry out an experiment in which he injected mice with nonvirulent, R pneumococci, derived by mutation from a type I S strain, together with dead (therefore also nonvirulent) type II S pneumococci. To his surprise, not only did the mice die but he isolated live type II S pneumococci from them. To him that meant something from the dead type II bacteria had been transferred to the R bacteria, derived from type I S, and had converted them to type II S bacteria. He called the phenomenon *transformation.*

Avery read the report of Griffith's experiments in 1928 and was very interested but not quite convinced at first. A young associate, Martin Dawson, repeated Griffith's experiments in great detail and confirmed the results. Now Avery accepted transformation as a real phenomenon and set out to find the nature of the substance that was responsible, which he called *transforming principle.* Later, Dawson was able to bring about transformation in the test tube by simply adding heat-killed type II pneumococci to a growing culture of R pneumococci derived from type I. This procedure made it much easier than the injection of bacteria into mice to test for transformation.

Colin MacLeod, a young Canadian physician joined Avery's laboratory in 1934. Over the subsequent years he and Avery carried out many experiments on the purification of the transforming principle that led to the realization that it did not consist of polysaccharide, protein, or ribonucleic acid (RNA). There were indications that it might consist of DNA. In 1941, MacLeod left Avery's laboratory to become chairman of the Microbiology Department at New York University School of Medicine. In the same year, Maclyn McCarty, another young physician arrived at the Rockefeller Institute and continued MacLeod's work. He continued the purification of the transforming principle and obtained the highest frequency of transformation with a preparation that consisted only of DNA. An enzyme that destroyed DNA also destroyed transforming activity. Thus, within 2 years, the transforming principle was definitely shown to be DNA. Unexpectedly, the factor transmitting the genetic information for the deadly capsule was in DNA.

In 1944 the publication of the work on the transforming principle caused great excitement in the scientific community but it also raised a good deal of skepticism. One of the chief critics was one of my advisers for graduate work, Alfred Mirsky. He had collaborated previously with Avery's group and had contributed to demonstrating that DNA was contained in the transforming principle. Now, he became doubtful that DNA by itself could be the genetic material. From what is said in Chapter 3 about the chemical nature of DNA, it had a monotonous structure of four repeated molecules, consisting of two purines called adenine and guanine, and two pyrimidines called thymine and cytosine, which did not provide enough variation to account for the differences seen among genes. Mirsky had studied the chemistry of nuclei and found that they contained proteins in addition to DNA. To him, proteins were much more likely candidates than DNA for determining the specificity of different genes. Mirsky was very persistent in his skepticism and his repeated public attacks on the validity of Avery's conclusions contributed to the long delay in the acceptance of DNA as the genetic substance.

By the time I finished my graduate work in 1946, it was certainly recognized that DNA had a fundamental role in heredity, although what role it played was not quite clear. My advisor, T. Dobzhansky, believed that pneumococcal DNA acted as a mutagenic agent. In the end it took another 10 years before it was universally accepted that genes consisted of DNA. Yet, the studies on the transforming principle had a decisive influence in channeling the efforts of research workers. Today, the work of the Avery Laboratory stands as a milestone in the history of molecular genetics.

The person who tried to deal with Mirsky's objections was Rollin Hotchkiss. He had joined Avery in 1946 and took over the laboratory after Avery's retirement in 1948. He was very well suited to fulfill this task: he was a very thorough, imaginative, and persistent investigator with a profound knowledge of biochemistry. His appearance and manner seemed to hide his sharp and penetrating intelligence. He spoke slowly and hesitatingly, ruminating each sentence. He had a dreamy expression on his face and, with his tousled hair, he gave the impression of being sleepy. Emerging through this exterior, his profound remarks often appeared all the more startling.

Hotchkiss kept on patiently purifying the transforming DNA until a point was reached in 1950 at which the protein content of his preparation was at most 0.02% of the total material. Yet the preparation was fully active in transformation. He also showed that his preparation could be inactivated by a crystalline, a very pure preparation of a DNA-destroying enzyme. At this point his critics accepted that the transformation of the capsular type was brought about by DNA alone. Hotchkiss then went on to show that his transforming DNA could transmit other genetic traits, such as resistance to streptomycin and penicillin and the ability to ferment certain sugars, such as mannitol. This indicated that many, if not all, genes of pneumococci were contained in the transforming DNA. It was then shown that transformation with DNA could occur with another disease-producing bacterium, *Hemophilus influenzae.* It thus became widely accepted that transformation was a general method for transferring genes contained in DNA from one bacterium to another.

As mentioned, a major theoretical obstacle to the acceptance of DNA as the genetic material was that the structure of DNA, proposed in 1931 by the Rockefeller Institute chemist Levene was too monotonous for the observed variety of genes. For example, one would expect that the gene responsible for streptomycin resistance would be different from the gene responsible for mannitol fermentation. However, if Levene's theory were correct, there would be no variation between these different genes. Hotchkiss was skeptical about the validity of Levene's hypothesis and began to investigate the constitution of DNA with the aim of more accurately identifying the structure of DNA. He used the more refined method of paper chromatography for measuring the four bases—adenine, thymine, guanine, and cytosine—present in DNA. This method had not been available to Levene. At the time of Hotchkiss' attempts, the same approach was used by the biochemist Erwin Chargaff at Columbia University. Although Hotchkiss obtained interesting preliminary results, he realized that Chargaff had superior expertise for this task and stopped his investigations. As he stated, "When I discovered that Chargaff's laboratory was developing their qualitative chromatography also into quantitative analysis, I retired from that field to do more biological things, after describing my methods for analyzing base mixtures." This attitude was indicative of his genuine practice of putting the progress of the work ahead of himself.

Chargaff, a native of Vienna, had joined the faculty of the Biochemistry Department at Columbia Medical School in 1935. Besides being an excellent biochemist, he was a broadly cultured person with a sharp wit. In appearance and manner he gave the impression of a European intellectual, clean shaven and with a somewhat forbidding expression on his face. The breadth of his interest can be realized from a book he published in 1986 entitled, *Serious Questions. An ABC of Skeptical Reflections.* This is a series of short essays, arranged in alphabetical order and ranging from "Amateurs" to "Zauberflöte."

At the beginning of World War II Chargaff received a contract with the Army Medical Service to study Rickettsia, the causative agent of typhus fever. In the early 1940s, he worked toward isolating the nucleic acids of these small organisms. By the time he had isolated the nucleic acids in 1944, the paper of Avery, MacLeod, and McCarty was published and Chargaff read it with great interest. In fact, he became so interested that he decided to devote his laboratory work completely to the study of nucleic acids. Thus, he was an ideal candidate to continue the pursuit of clarifying the structure of DNA with more accuracy.

Chargaff engaged a young and able Swiss biochemist, Ernst Vischer, to measure the amounts of the four bases in different preparations of DNA and to determine their ratios. According to the monotonous theory of Levene, they were 1:1:1:1. However, Chargaff and Vischer showed that for calf thymus DNA, they were 1.7 adenine:1.6 thymine:1.2 guanine:1.0 cytosine. For other DNA preparations, they also found deviations from the 1:1:1:1 ratio. Thus, Chargaff disproved Levene's theory.

If DNA is the genetic material, one would expect that the base ratios for DNA from different species would be different given that they are genetically different. However, the ratios from different tissues of the *same* organism should be the same given that they have the same genetic constitution. This is exactly what Chargaff and Vischer observed.

In the course of studying DNA preparations from many different species they noticed a curious regularity. In all of them, the amount of adenine was equal to the amount of thymine, and the amount of guanine was equal to the amount of cytosine. Chargaff mulled over these unexpected regularities but he was unable to find an explanation for the puzzling phenomenon. Later these equalities became known as Chargaff's Rules and they played an important part in working out the structure of DNA.

Ultimately the studies of Hotchkiss and Chargaff paved the way for an experiment that did contribute further to the acceptance of DNA as the genetic material. This experiment was carried out at Cold Spring Harbor by Hershey, the third member of the original phage triumvirate, and his collaborator, Martha Chase. Although the most reticent of the three, the other two being Luria and Delbrück, he was a deep thinker and came up with many original ideas and experiments.

In the late 1940s, it became known that the bacteriophages studied by the phage group consisted of protein and DNA. Under the electron microscope, bacteriophages looked like little tadpoles with heads and tails. When these creatures infected a bacterium, they attached themselves to the outside by their tail and injected some of the contents into the bacterium, like hypodermic needles would. Subsequently, multiplication occurred, giving rise to a crop of several hundred new bacteriophages. The bacterium lysed and the new bacteriophages were released. The question was: What was injected into the bacterium? Was it protein or DNA, or both?

Hershey and Chase attacked this question experimentally by using radioactive compounds to label protein and DNA separately. They labeled protein with radioactive sulfur and DNA with radioactive phosphorus. By infecting bacteria with labeled bacteriophages and analyzing the radioactivity of the bacteriophages that were released, they found that mainly the DNA entered the bacteria and most of the protein remained on the outside. The genetic continuity of the bacteriophages was provided by DNA.

The Hershey-Chase experiment attracted wide attention. In particular, the results of this experiment convinced a young American biologist, James Watson working in Denmark whose main interest had been the nature of genes, that his mission was to work out the structure of DNA. Shortly after digesting the full implications of the Hershey-Chase experiment, he left Denmark for England determined to carry out that mission.

Watson was a lanky young man, diffident and bored in manner except when regarding a topic that interested him. He had been a precocious student having entered the University of Chicago at the age of 15 years old. Before that, he had been one of the Chicago Quiz Kids in a popular radio show. He had a passionate interest in ornithology and was an expert bird watcher. After graduating from the University of Chicago, he began graduate work at the University of Indiana. He was attracted by Luria's work on bacteriophage genetics and did his PhD thesis work with him on the effects of X-rays on the development of bacteriophages. In this way, he became the youngest member of the Phage Group.

After receiving his PhD degree at the age of 22, Watson went to Europe to broaden his education. He studied the metabolism of *E. coli* infected with bacteriophages in the laboratory of Ole Maaloe in Copenhagen but the biochemical orientation of the laboratory did not appeal to him. It did not deal with the nature of the gene, which was his central interest. In the spring of 1951, he attended a meeting in Naples where he heard a talk by the British crystallographer Maurice Wilkins on the structure of DNA. Wilkins showed an X-ray picture of the crystalline form of DNA. Suddenly Watson became excited and decided on the spur of the moment to switch fields. Unable to establish contact with Wilkins who worked at King's College, London, he went to the Cavendish Laboratory in Cambridge, the next best place for his purpose. There he met Francis Crick. Their meeting, at the right time and the right place, was of historic importance (Fig. 7–1).

The Cavendish Laboratory was devoted to the study of the structure of large

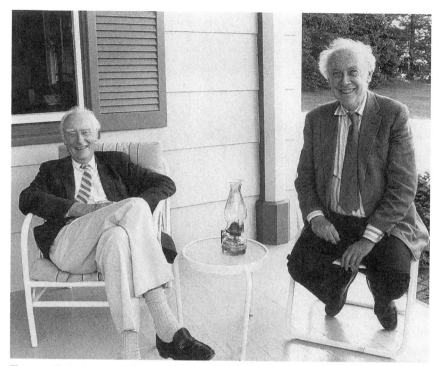

Figure 7–1. A recent photograph of Francis Crick (*left*) and James Watson (*right*) at Cold Spring Harbor. [Courtesy of Cold Spring Harbor Laboratory Library Archives.]

molecules, especially proteins, by X-ray crystallography. It housed several brilliant investigators who were engaged in determining the position of atoms within protein molecules from X-ray photographs of crystals. With this method they could establish the three-dimensional structure of these molecules. They were aided greatly in this endeavor by the construction of molecular models made of metal. These helped to interpret the structures derived from X-ray photographs.

Watson and Crick shared a burning interest in determining the structure of DNA by X-ray crystallography. They agreed to collaborate on the project. Moreover, they decided to limit their efforts to model building and to use the X-ray crystallography data of other investigators, notably Maurice Wilkins and his colleague Rosalind Franklin at King's College in London, for the construction of their models.

Crick was in many ways the opposite of Watson. Whereas Watson was often moody and silent, Crick was extroverted, cheerful, and enthusiastic, and always talking. He was about as tall as Watson, but looked slightly more robust. He could talk for hours on end, always coming up with new ideas. In 1954, I recall, during an 8-hour ride in my car, going from New York City to New Hampshire to attend a conference, he never stopped talking once. But, it was absolutely engaging and exciting as he was in the thick of exploring a new theory to be discussed later in Chapter 9. In such circumstances, it is always fascinating to observe Crick's ability to articulate his most complex and sophisticated ideas as if they were merely simple and commonplace thoughts. This has never been the product of false modesty but is more a product of his natural tendency to be open and readily make his ideas accessible to others.

Crick was originally trained as a physicist, but he decided after World War II, during which he had done war service for the British Admiralty, to switch to biology. Like other physicists at the time, he seems to have been disillusioned by the course physics was taking, possibly because of the development of the atomic bomb. Shortly after I met him in 1954 I asked him why he switched from physics to biology. In his cheerful manner, he replied: "Oh, I read this fascinating book on biochemistry, called *The Dynamic State of Body Constituents* and I found that I was so good at explaining it to my fellow physicists that I decided that biology must be my calling." Although there may have been other reasons for the switch, this sounded plausible and fitting with his personality.

His first studies in biology were on the effects of ingested iron on cells in tissue culture but he found this work uninteresting. He then went to the Cavendish Laboratory to apprentice himself to the crystallographer Max Perutz, who was in the beginning stages of working out the structure of hemoglobin, for which he was later awarded a Nobel Prize. Under Perutz's guidance he learned both the practical and theoretical elements of X-ray crystallography of large molecules. When he met Watson in 1951, he already had 2 years' experience in this field.

Watson and Crick hit it off from the start. They complemented each other in scientific background as well as in temperament. While Crick was an inexhaustible source of ideas for the possible structure of molecules, Watson helped him to refine his models by serving as a challenging sounding board. They were free spirits not tied down by conventions and they were uninhibited in the pursuit of their ideas. They were critical of each other but in a constructive manner, which helped them to avoid dead ends in their investigations. Above all, they were constantly drawn together by their common goal to work out the structure of DNA.

In 1951, Perutz and the other investigators at the Cavendish Laboratory were trying to determine the backbone structure of protein molecules using model-building to find a structure that best fitted the X-ray crystallographic data. They were frustrated in being unable to find a fitting structure. Success came from another source, the laboratory of Linus Pauling in Pasadena. His model building led to the correct structure, a type of helix called an α helix. Grudgingly, the workers at Cambridge had to admit that Pauling single handedly had beaten them to the draw. But Pauling had not applied his helix model-building method to DNA—yet.

Watson and Crick started their work on the structure of DNA in 1951. The task of building a model that fit all the data was arduous and often frustrating. It took 2 years with many failures before they arrived at a fitting structure. This structure consisted of two DNA strands intertwined into a Double Helix with pairs of bases holding the strands together like the rungs of a ladder.

The arrangement was such that adenine in one strand was always connected to thymine in the other strand by weak chemical bonds called hydrogen bonds and, in the same way, guanine in one strand was always connected to cytosine in the other strand. Because of this, one could finally visualize in a tangible manner how genes replicate and act.

These fixed structural relationships that were shown by their double helix had been predicted by Chargaff's Rules, of which Watson and Crick had not been aware until they were told about them by Chargaff during a visit to Cambridge. They were overjoyed by the unexpected support for their model. Chargaff however, must have had bitter feelings afterwards. Perhaps if he had been less restrained and more audacious, he might have come up with a model for DNA himself. This certainly would have given greater prominence to his role in the elucidation of the structure of DNA. Nevertheless, Chargaff's Rules were a great contribution to the development of molecular genetics and they stand as a benchmark on the road to the double helix.

Watson has given a vivid account of his work with Crick in the best-selling book *The Double Helix*. With unrestrained frankness he described their ups and downs and their anxiety about the progress of the other investigators, especially Wilkins and Franklin in London and Pauling lurking in Pasadena. They were deadly afraid that the latter's genius would lead him to the correct structure before they arrived there. This fear, together with their awareness of the prize at stake, contributed greatly to their persistence to solve the structure of DNA.

The Watson-Crick double helix structure was a crowning achievement. By itself, it did not *prove* that DNA alone was the genetic material, but there were intriguing features of the double helix that made it plausible that its structure was sufficient to account for all the properties of genes. Previously there had always been a shroud of mystery about gene activities. It was a common feeling among geneticists that genes were very complicated biochemically and that it would take many years, if ever, before their activities could be unraveled. The double helix, with a single stroke, dispelled these gloomy predictions. Within a short time most people accepted the notion that DNA was synonymous with genes. Thus, all the previous efforts to demonstrate that genes consisted only of DNA, starting from Avery's work and up to the Hershey-Chase experiment, were vindicated. The double helix heralded the Golden Age of molecular genetics.

The ability of genes to replicate could finally be explained by the double helix structure. To illustrate how the replicative function could be achieved, in their first publication on the structure of DNA in 1953, Watson and Crick stated: "It has not escaped our notice that the specific pairing (between complementary bases) we have postulated immediately suggests a possible copying mechanism for the genetic material."

In such a mechanism the two DNA strands would become separated, with the breaking of the hydrogen bonds joining the complementary bases along the double helix ladder. Each strand would then form a template for the formation of a complementary strand. All that was necessary was for each base in the DNA strand to pair with a free complementary base. After that, the newly laid down bases would be joined to each other, forming the complementary strand. In this way, an exact replica of the double helix molecule would be produced, as illustrated in Figure 7–2.

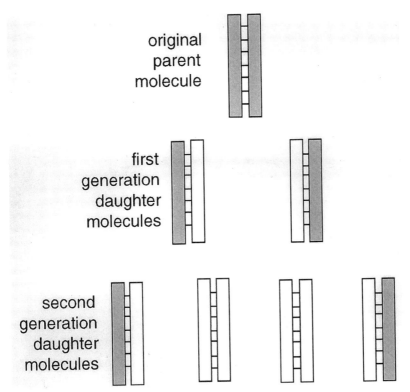

original
parent
molecule

first
generation
daughter
molecules

second
generation
daughter
molecules

FIGURE 7–2. Schematic presentation of semiconservative replication of double-stranded DNA. The shaded bars are the two strands of the original double helix, the white bars represent newly-synthesized DNA. The cross bars join complementary bases in the two strands.

The Watson and Crick proposal for replication was very plausible but it needed experimental evidence to prove its validity. This was achieved in 1958, 5 years after the publication of their proposal. Two young investigators at Caltech, M. Meselson and F.M. Stahl demonstrated that the mechanism of semi-conservative replication occurs in nature (see Fig. 7–2). They did this in a brilliant experiment by using isotopically labeled bases to distinguish between the parental double helix molecule and the two newly replicated double helix molecules.

Crick did not rest on his laurels for having elucidated the structure of DNA and its consequences in replication for long, but was already pursuing in 1953 the next job that lay ahead, i.e., how the double helix of DNA could determine the structure of protein molecules. He knew that this was going to be much more difficult to visualize than the process of replication. The relevant facts were that DNA molecules consisted of long double helical chains in which adenine-thymine and guanine-cytosine base pairs were arranged in a definite sequence, and that, in a similar fashion, protein molecules consisted of long chains of amino acids, also arranged in a definite sequence. These facts were the first to define the science of genetics at a level from which the action of genes, as determined by the structure of DNA, could be visualized. It was assumed that the specific sequence of base pairs in DNA somehow coded for a specific sequence of amino acids, just as signals generated by a television camera code for a picture on a television screen.

III

HOW GENES
DETERMINE
PROTEIN STRUCTURE
1953–1965

I N 1953, after the structure of DNA was solved, the central problem in biology became that of the gene-controlled synthesis of proteins in the living cell. How did a sequence of nucleotides in a DNA molecule constituting a gene determine the structure of a protein molecule? The problem was addressed in three ways. The first was the work of biochemists who investigated systematically the steps involved in protein synthesis starting from the amino acid building blocks. The second was the work of geneticists using classical methods of genetic analysis to gain information about gene action at the molecular level. The third was based on theories of coding and was new in biology. In interdependent ways, the three approaches brought about the elucidation of protein synthesis as determined by the information contained in DNA.

Three discoveries can be singled out that tied DNA to protein synthesis. The first involved the identification of what Crick called *adaptors*, molecules that were required for connecting the message coming from DNA in the nucleus to the protein-synthesizing machinery in the cytoplasm. In 1956, a group of biochemists in Boston discovered small RNA molecules that were required for protein synthesis and whose activities matched the postulated function of Crick's adaptor molecules. They called them transfer RNAs (tRNAs).

The second discovery was the recognition of an unstable RNA called messenger RNA that was copied from one of the DNA strands of the double helix in the nucleus and was then transported to the protein-synthesizing machinery in the cytoplasm. There the amino acids were lined up according to the genetic code transmitted to the synthesizing machinery and joined together to form a protein molecule.

The third discovery was the deciphering of the genetic code contained in messenger RNA. This feat was carried out initially by two young biochemists at the National Institutes of Health in Bethesda and was further substantiated by biochemists and geneticists. It revealed the arrangement of nucleotide bases in DNA that were responsible for determining each amino acid in a protein molecule.

The overall process of information flow became known as the Central Dogma:

$$DNA \rightarrow RNA \rightarrow Protein,$$

with DNA being the primary informational macromolecule.

8

Building a Theoretical Framework
for Gene Action

━━━━━━━━━━━━━━━━
━━━━━━━━━━━━━━━━
━━━━━━━━━━━━━━━━

I N 1953, Crick began to construct a general theory for the mechanism of gene action in the control of protein synthesis. In his delightful book *What Mad Pursuit* there is a chapter entitled "Theory in Molecular Biology." There he justifies his theoretical approach by saying that problems like the mechanism of gene action may not be solved by theoretical approaches alone, but that a general theoretical framework will be helpful in guiding the directions that experiments might take. The history of molecular genetics has given ample proof of the validity of Crick's attitude. It should be said, however, that Crick was unusual among theoreticians in that he was always very careful to take into account the restrictions imposed on his theories by experimental facts.

With the double helix in view, Crick built his theory on the foundation of what was known about protein synthesis. This subject had been studied during the 1930s and 1940s mainly in the laboratories of Torbjörn Caspersson, a microscopist in Sweden, and Jean Brachet, an embryologist in Belgium. Caspersson had developed a quartz-lensed microscope that could locate nucleic acids precisely in different parts of an individual living cell. He took advantage of the fact that nucleic acids absorb ultraviolet light that is transmitted through quartz. The two types of nucleic acid could then be differentiated by the previously mentioned Feulgen reaction that stains DNA but not RNA. Brachet in Brussels had also developed a staining mixture for nucleic acids that could distinguish between DNA and RNA. This mixture, consisting of the two dyes, pyronin and methyl green, stained DNA green and RNA red. A mixture of DNA and RNA stained blue. The mixture could be resolved by treatment with the enxyme ribonuclease that digested RNA but not DNA. After such treatment the blue-staining area now stained green like DNA.

Caspersson and Brachet studied the tissues and organs of diverse plants and animals during different stages of their development. From these studies they arrived at the following general conclusions: (1) The intracellular localization of DNA and RNA is different. DNA is found only in the nucleus whereas RNA is present mainly in the cytoplasm with a small amount in the nucleus. (2) In a particular species the amount of DNA per nucleus remains constant whereas the amount of RNA varies considerably from one tissue to another. (3) There is a strong correlation between the quantity of RNA in a cell and its capacity to synthesize proteins.

The distribution of RNA within a cell was studied by Brachet and by Albert Claude at the Rockefeller Institute in New York City. They separated the chemically different cellular components by ultracentrifugation. They found that most of the RNA was associated with minute particles, which they called microsomes. Later these particles were more clearly defined and named ribosomes. Presumably protein synthesis was associated with ribosomes.

Crick used the general picture generated by these studies for the construction of his model of protein synthesis. He assumed that genes contained in the DNA of the nucleus were copied into RNA. It was easy to see how a gene, consisting of a stretch of DNA, would make an RNA copy, in the same way as it makes a DNA copy during replication. This RNA would be transported to the cytoplasm where it would become associated with a protein to form a ribosome. Crick called this RNA *messenger RNA*. He assumed that there was a separate messenger RNA for each gene. In that way each ribosome would carry out the synthesis of one protein.

Crick's first question was concerned with the way genetic information was stored in the double helix of DNA. He was wondering how a sequence consisting of the four different bases present in DNA (adenine, guanine, cytosine, thymine = A,G,C,T) could be translated into a sequence consisting of the 20 different amino acids known to occur in protein molecules. This problem is similar to the Morse Code in which different combinations of dots and dashes are translated into the 26 letters of the alphabet. Because of this similarity Crick named the different combinations of bases coding for different amino acids in protein molecules the *Genetic Code*. The idea of such a code was not new. It was first proposed in 1945 by the physicist Erwin Schrödinger, in a book entitled, *What is Life?* This book was read widely and it convinced several physicists that there were interesting and provocative problems in biology, especially in genetics. In 1950, Sir Cyril Hinshelwood, Professor of Physical

Chemistry at Oxford, published some speculations along similar lines. A more concrete version of a code was proposed by Alexander Dounce in 1952.

In 1953 Crick met Sidney Brenner. The latter had grown up in South Africa and had received his early education at the University of Witwatersrand in Johannesburg where he studied medicine. He had then come to Oxford and enrolled for a PhD degree with Hinshelwood who had become interested in biological problems and started Brenner on a project involving bacteriophages. Brenner was fascinated by molecular genetics. He and Crick hit it off with each other immediately and became long-time associates. In 1954 Brenner went back to South Africa to fulfill some obligations but returned to England after 2 years and settled in Cambridge where he shared an office with Crick.

A set of adjacent bases coding for one amino acid was called a *codon*, a term invented by Brenner. An immediate question was how many bases there are in a codon. With two bases in a codon, there are only 16 possible codons (4×4), which is not enough to code for the 20 amino acids known to be in proteins. With three bases per codon, there are 64 different possibilities ($4 \times 4 \times 4$), which is more than sufficient to cover 20 amino acids. Better too many than not enough. Crick and Brenner concluded that most likely each codon consisted of three bases.

At this point, a twist in the coding problem occurred when Watson and Crick received a letter from George Gamow, a Russian-born American physicist who had become famous as the proponent of the Big Bang Theory. He was also the author of a popular series of books about science in which a Mr. Tomkins was the main character. Gamow had been intrigued by the paper about the structure of DNA that had appeared in the journal *Nature*. In pondering over a possible code, he had conceived of the idea that the DNA structure by itself, without the intervention of RNA, could act as a template for the assembly of amino acids to form a protein. He noticed that because of different local arrangements of bases, there were 20 different kinds of cavities in the DNA structure. Given that it was known that there are 20 different amino acids in proteins, he assumed that there was one type of cavity for each amino acid. Subsequently, Gamow submitted a paper for publication describing his scheme in which the fictitious Tomkins was listed as a second author. Unfortunately the editor was familiar with Gamow's books and Tomkin's name was removed before publication.

Crick and Watson considered Gamow's proposal very carefully. It had some attractive features but there were too many other features that did not fit. In the end, Crick, during a stay at the Brooklyn Polytechnic Institute in New York during the winter of 1953–1954, managed to disprove all possible versions of Gamow's code. He used the protein sequence data then available and assumed that the code was *universal*, that is, was the same in all living organisms. Later the assumption was shown to be correct.

One of the features of Gamow's proposal was that the code was overlapping. To illustrate what this means, let us consider a six-base sequence, AATCGA. In an overlapping code, the maximum number of codons would be four: AAT, ATC, TCG, and CGA, whereas in a nonoverlapping code, it would only be two: AAT and CGA. From an examination of the known protein sequences, Crick concluded that an overlapping code was unlikely. The argument against an overlapping code was sharpened later by Brenner after his return from South Africa. On the basis of the number of different dipeptide sequences (a dipeptide consists of two amino acids linked through a peptide bond) in known protein sequences (70) and the theoretically expected number of possible dipeptide sequences in an overlapping code (64), he concluded that all overlapping triplet codes were impossible.

As an aside, a good example of the great utility of chemical methods for genetic considerations was the development of a sequencing method for proteins. This was achieved in 1951 by the biochemist Fred Sanger, a colleague of Crick who received a Nobel prize for this work. He later developed a method for sequencing nucleic acids (see p. 132), which is of immeasurable value for genetic studies. For this work he received a second Nobel prize.

Crick met Gamow for the first time in the fall of 1953 in Brooklyn. Vittorio Luzzati, an Italian crystallographer with whom Crick shared an office, described the meeting as follows: "They were both shouting. Crick and Gamow. They were in excellent spirits, not quarreling at all. Enthusiastic about what they were discussing."

Gamow was extremely extroverted. Later he founded an organization called the RNA Tie Club. There were 20 members, one for each of the 20 amino acids. Besides the RNA tie, designed by Gamow and produced by a haberdasher in Oxford, each member was to wear a tie pin that carried the three-letter abbreviation of his assigned amino acid. The purpose of the Tie Club was to encourage discussion and to circulate papers that were more speculative than their authors would risk in formal publications.

At that time Crick began to think about the necessity of having what he called adaptors to line up on the ribosome the sequence of bases in the messenger RNA with the proper sequence of amino acids in the protein. He could not envisage how a messenger RNA could by itself provide a direct template for the 20 different amino acids. What was needed were 20 different adaptor molecules that on one side could combine with a codon of the messenger RNA and on the other side with a specific amino acid. The adaptor molecules would contain an "anticodon" site to combine with the codon and another site to combine with a specific amino acid. After forming a bond with its amino acid each adaptor molecule would find its codon on the messenger RNA. The amino acids present on adjacent adaptor molecules would combine with each other to become assembled into a protein molecule. Crick submitted his first publication on the Adaptor Hypothesis to the RNA Tie Club.

The Adaptor Hypothesis was the main topic of the animated conversation we had during the previously mentioned car trip from New York to New Hampshire in 1954. There were three of us in the car, Crick, myself, and my associate Michael Yarmolinsky. I remember how Crick was considering various substances as possible candidates for his postulated adaptors. One type of molecule that seemed to appeal to him was a sugar molecule. He did not consider nucleic acids because he thought they were too large. As we shall see in the next chapter, his concern was unfounded and the adaptors turned out to be small RNA molecules. At any rate, the discussion was very lively and exciting. I was not aware at the time that I was witnessing the birth of one of the key hypotheses of molecular genetics.

An important implication of the Adaptor Hypothesis was that it liberated the Genetic Code from the structural constraints of the amino acids having to combine in a specific fashion with messenger RNA. Each amino acid only had to combine with its adaptor. The latter would then find its place in the messenger RNA. These anticodon fittings, like the genetic code itself, had probably originated millions of years ago and had been maintained during the course of evolution.

With a nonoverlapping three-letter (triplet) code established, the next question to be considered was how many of the 64 possible triplets actually coded for an amino acid and for the identity of the amino acid. These questions, although identified by the theoretical approach, could only be answered experimentally. They had to await the work of biochemists, as is discussed in Chapter 11. It was not until 1965 that the details of the complete genetic code were worked out.

Another aspect of Crick's scheme that begged for biochemical verification was the notion that there should be a ribosome for each gene and its corresponding messenger RNA. Assuming that there are 20,000 genes this would imply the formation of 20,000 different ribosomes. This seemed to create an unwieldy situation in the cytoplasm. As is discussed later, in Chapter 10 the biochemical reality turned out to be much more manageable.

Overall, Crick's theoretical scheme was a masterful plan for the steps of gene action in protein synthesis. It consisted of two separate stages. First the coded message in DNA was transcribed into the messenger RNA. This RNA moved from the nucleus into the cytoplasm where it was incorporated into ribosomes. Second, the message contained in messenger RNA was translated on the ribosomes with the aid of adaptors into the amino acid chains constituting protein molecules. As is discussed in the following 3 chapters, this overall scheme served as a most useful guide to direct the research efforts of both geneticists and biochemists, in spite of the changes that had to be made along the way. Without having Crick's theoretical guidance available it would have taken much longer to achieve the final picture of gene action described in Chapter 14. Crick's sentiment about the value of theory in scientific research, mentioned at the beginning of this chapter, was validated by history.

9

Biochemical Identification
of Adaptors

DURING 1953, while Crick was busy in Cambridge constructing his model of gene action, two groups of biochemists at the Massachusetts General Hospital in Boston were working on the steps of protein synthesis starting from the level of amino acids. Eventually their studies would lead to the identification of Crick's adaptors. However, in 1953 they were not aware of Crick's efforts and they would have been surprised to learn that within a short time they would meet him and become involved in a joint enterprise. In this chapter we see how this meeting came about and how it led to the chemical identification of the adapter molecules.

The first group was headed by Fritz Lipmann (Fig. 9–1). Originally trained as a physician in Germany, he had become interested in biochemistry and started an apprenticeship at the Kaiser Wilhelm Institute in Berlin in the laboratory of Otto Meyerhof. It was there that he began to realize the importance of phosphate in the reactions that supply the energy for biosynthetic reactions. He eventually formulated the concept of a universal chemical energy source in the form of a substance called adenosine triphosphate (ATP), which served as energy-donating currency. Adenosine triphosphate consists of the nucleic acid base adenine linked to the sugar ribose, which in turn is linked to three phosphate molecules in a row (see Fig. 9–2). Lipmann called the bonds between the three phosphate molecules in ATP *high-energy bonds* and denoted them

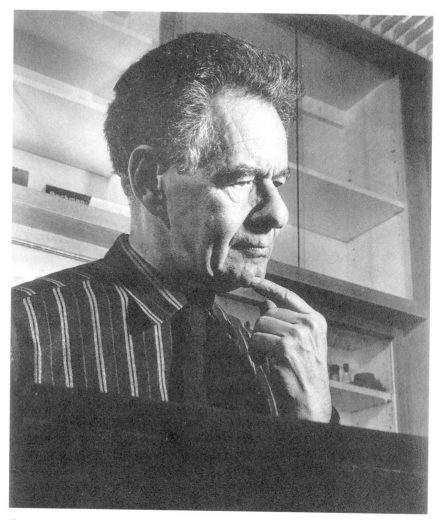

FIGURE 9–1. Fritz Lipmann in a pensive mood. [Courtesy of Freda Hall-Lipman.]

by a squiggle (~). This notion of Lipmann became a unifying concept in biochemistry.

In 1931, Lipmann came to the Rockefeller Institute for 2 years to work with Phoebus Levene. He returned to Europe, but because of the Nazi regime in Germany chose to live in Denmark. He returned once more to the United States, this time permanently, in 1939. He set up his own laboratory in 1941 at the Massachusetts General Hospital. At that time he wrote a review entitled, "Metabolic Generation and Utilization of Phosphate Bond Energy," which attracted wide attention, and also marked the beginning of his interest in protein

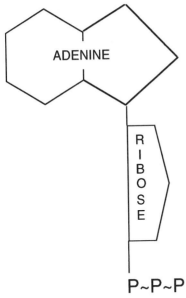

FIGURE 9–2. Schematic presentation of the chemical structure of adenosine triphosphate.

synthesis. He assumed that in the formation of a peptide bond between two amino acids, one of these had to react with ATP and acquire a phosphate molecule, to become activated for the subsequent joining with the other amino acid.

To study how ATP is utilized in peptide bond formation, Lipmann used model compounds that contained only one peptide bond. Protein molecules contain many peptide bonds between different amino acids arranged in a definite order, but the use of proteins would complicate the study of peptide bond formation. One such model compound was pantothenic acid, whose synthesis I had studied in Davis' laboratory. Lipmann had shown that pantothenic acid is the major constituent of coenzyme A, a coenzyme which he had discovered in the 1940s. A coenzyme is a substance that combines with an enzyme to enable it to carry out a specific function. In the case of coenzyme A, this function is called acetylation, the addition of acetic acid in the formation of metabolites. Acetylation reactions are frequent and play an important role in metabolism. Lipmann was awarded a Nobel Prize in 1953 for his discovery of coenzyme A.

Since my work on the enzyme that makes pantothenic acid was closely related to Lipmann's work on coenzyme A, I was eager to work on the mechanism of this enzymatic reaction in his laboratory. It would give me some excellent training in biochemistry. In 1950 I heard him speak in New York about his work on coenzyme A. It was then that I gathered enough courage to approach him and tell him about my work on pantothenic acid. I asked him if I could work in his laboratory and was very pleased when he invited me to come to Boston for a year.

In 1950 I was not aware of the significance of the pantothenate-synthesizing enzyme for the study of peptide bond formation and it was only after I arrived in Boston in 1952 that I found out about that aspect of Lipmann's interest in my enzyme. By that time I had learned that the formation of the peptide bond in pantothenic acid requires ATP. My first task was to find out which of the two precursors of pantothenic acid, beta-alanine or pantoic acid reacted with ATP to become activated. My first results indicated that the enzyme itself, not the two precursors, reacted with ATP. This seemed strange but it pleased Lipmann that the enzyme itself could become the source of the energy for peptide bond formation. After returning to New York in 1954 I continued the purification of the pantothenate synthesizing enzyme in my own laboratory at New York University. It turned out that my result in Lipmann's laboratory had been spurious because of contamination with another enzyme in my extracts. In collaboration with my associate Michael Yarmolinsky and Daniel Koshland of the Brookhaven National Laboratory, who supplied us with O^{18} for isotopic labeling experiments, I demonstrated with a highly purified enzyme preparation that it was pantoic acid that became activated. The activated compound was pantoyl ~ adenylic acid, which has a high-energy phosphate bond between pantoic acid and the one phosphate group present in adenylic acid.

Since pantothenic acid, although important in its own right as a constituent of coenzyme A, was used here as a model peptide, the next question was: Is the activating mechanism of pantothenic acid synthesis the same as the one occurring in peptide bond formation in proteins? This question was of great interest one floor above Lipmann's laboratory to Paul Zamecnik, the head of the second group and his associate Mahlon Hoagland.

Zamecnik, who had a medical background had originally set up his laboratory to carry out research on cancer. His idea was to study protein synthesis in normal and malignant tissues for the purpose of finding differences that would be useful for the understanding of cancer and the design of anticancer drugs. He began to realize that in order to do this work he needed to have a good system for studying protein synthesis. He and his associates gradually developed a cell-free system prepared from rat livers in which they could demonstrate the occurrence of protein synthesis. They used radioactive amino acids as tracers and followed their incorporation into proteins as a measure of protein synthesis.

Hoagland, who had joined Zamecnik after spending a year in Lipmann's laboratory, was familiar with the method I had developed for the demonstration of pantoyl ~ adenylic acid. He found, using this method, that in their rat-liver preparations that were active in protein synthesis, addition of amino acids and ATP led to the formation of aminoacyl ~ adenylates, analogous to the formation of pantoyl ~ adenylate in pantothenate synthesis. Thus, the mechanism of activation for the formation of the peptide bond in protein synthesis was the same as the mechanism of amino acid activation in pantothenic acid synthesis. However, as we shall see, in the case of protein synthesis the activated amino acids do not form a peptide bond immediately, but only after a circuitous route of intermediate reactions. Further work by Hoagland and in Lipmann's laboratory led to the recognition that there were many amino-acid activating enzymes, one for the activation of each of the 20 amino acids. They carry out the first step on the road to the formation of proteins.

In the case of proteins, in contrast to pantothenic acid, a question was posed by the specific array of amino acids in a protein: How does an activated amino acid find its proper neighbor in the protein chain? Lipmann was very puzzled by this question. He referred to the specific sequence of amino acids as *patternization*. In an article published in 1956 entitled, "Basic Biochemical Questions," he stated the problem as follows: "The energy requirement for patternization may be divided into (1) a well-defined caloric equivalent for the joining of the links in the backbone structure (i.e., peptide bond formation) and (2) an 'energy of position,' the directing into a specific order. The latter is biologically the most important. We meet here a novel situation, and its biochemical definition has no well-understood examples to fall back upon. The principle of 'patternization' has in fact become the meeting ground between biochemistry and genetics. To define the problem in all its facets, a fusion of biochemical and genetic principles will be needed."

What Lipmann referred to in his pronouncement as a novel situation was the translation of a specific sequence of bases in DNA into a specific sequence of amino acids in a protein. This was the same question posed by Crick and formulated by him as the genetic code. Lipmann was a classical biochemist without prior training in genetics and he was not familiar with the language of geneticists. But he seemed to have intuitively realized the implications of genes as determinants of the structure of proteins. This was typical of the broad insight he had into the biochemical processes in cells. This characteristic distinguished him from most other biochemists, whose outlook was more narrow, and who tended to confine themselves to one particular biochemical process. When Lipmann made a prediction about a biochemical reaction that he was studying, he was usually correct. I once witnessed an interview with a reporter in which he was asked about the secret of his success in working out biochemical processes. He smiled, and said: "Oh, I just follow my nose."

After the discovery of the amino acid activating enzymes present in the cytoplasm, Zamecnik and Hoagland were wondering where the peptide bond formation occurred. Was it in solution in the cytoplasm (also called the cytosol) or was it at the sites called ribosomes? There were also some indications that there might be another intermediary compound between the activation reaction and peptide bond formation.

The answer to these questions came when Zamecnik and Hoagland accidentally found that the activated amino acids reacted with an RNA, rather than another amino acid, to form a stable compound. This RNA was not ribosomal RNA, but a relatively small unknown RNA molecule, about 75 nucleotides in length, that was present in the cytosol. They called this RNA s-RNA for soluble RNA. In fact, there seemed to be many types of s-RNAs, at least one for each amino acid. Then Hoagland did a crucial experiment in which he demonstrated, using radioactive amino acids, that each amino acid was transferred from its s-RNA-amino acid compound to a growing protein molecule in the ribosomes. For this reason it was also called transfer RNA. It became clear that transfer RNA was a physical link between activated amino acids and their ordered incorporation into protein molecules. At last the postulated function of Crick's adaptors was demonstrated. A transfer RNA for alanine was discovered independently at this time by Robert Holley. Later he isolated this transfer RNA and determined its nucleotide sequence. For this work he was awarded a Nobel Prize in 1968.

The work of Hoagland and Zamecnik attracted the attention of Watson, Crick's old partner, who had by then taken an academic appointment at Harvard. Watson visited Hoagland and told him about Crick's adaptor hypothesis, which had not yet been published. It became clear to Hoagland that his transfer RNAs were Crick's adaptors. They were thought to combine on one end with an amino acid and on the other end, the anticodon site, with a codon in the messenger RNA in the ribosomes. Hoagland was pleased that he had confirmed Crick's prediction but he was also somewhat miffed for having been beaten to the draw. After all, here he was, a physician turned into an enterprising and enthusiastic biochemist who within a few years had made his way to the forefront of the exciting developments in protein synthesis. As he stated rather poetically: "A vision arose before me—we explorers sweating and slashing our way through a dense jungle, finally rewarded by the discovery of a beautiful long-lost temple—and looking up to see Crick, circling above our goal on gossamer wings of theory, gleefully pointing it out to us."

After Crick heard about Hoagland's results, he visited him in Boston in 1957 and invited him to come to Cambridge to carry out joint experiments. Hoagland accepted and spent the next academic year in Cambridge doing experiments with Zamecnik's cell-free system isolated from rat liver to further establish the role of transfer RNAs as intermediaries in protein synthesis. It was during this collaboration that Hoagland found Crick one morning, in the laboratory bent under a bench chasing a rat that was apparently eluding Crick's efforts to use its liver as a source of material for their biochemical experiments. This scene demonstrates the extent of the breakdown of the barrier between biochemists and genetically oriented theoreticians that had begun shortly after the unveiling of the double helix in 1953.

Hoagland's sojourn in Crick's laboratory was a link in the chain of developments that led from Lipmann's work on the amino acid activation by ATP for peptide bond synthesis to Hoagland's discovery of transfer RNA as an essential component of the protein synthesizing machinery, to Crick's postulate that there must be adaptors that transfer the information contained in the messenger RNA sequence to the alignment of amino acids in protein molecules. Just as the ribosome was the physical meeting ground for combining the coded message with amino acids, it was the meeting ground for theoretical geneticists and biochemists such as Crick and Hoagland to work out the steps of protein synthesis. One came from the level of DNA the other from the level of amino acids, the building blocks of protein.

10

The Elusive Messenger

AFTER the discovery of transfer RNAs and their role in protein synthesis, the theoretical framework that Crick was drawing for protein synthesis became more detailed. After forming aminoacyl adenylates, the amino acids were joined to transfer RNAs (adaptors), which in turn delivered them to the messenger RNA in the ribosomes. Lined up on the messenger RNA, the amino acids were joined to each other to form the protein molecules.

In a larger sense, the coded message, which had been copied from the DNA in the nucleus onto RNA, had to move from the nucleus through the nuclear membrane to the cytoplasm. There it would combine with ribosomal protein to form a ribosome. In this position it would supervise the making of a protein. While the transfer RNA that brought the amino acids to the ribosomes was clearly identified, the identification of the bulk RNA of the ribosomes with messenger RNA was still an assumption. Furthermore, it was only an assumption that each ribosome synthesized just one protein and that its RNA was the postulated messenger RNA copied from the DNA of the nuclear gene.

These assumptions began to bother Crick and his colleague Brenner. Although he was pleased with the overall picture, Crick realized there were some features that did not fit. At this time, ribosomes were being studied extensively and much was known about their constitution. Thus, it had been shown by biochemists that ribosomes contained only two RNAs of different sizes. Yet Crick and Brenner surmised that if these RNAs were the messenger RNAs, they would come in many different lengths, since protein molecules come in many different sizes. This and a number of other discrepancies suggested to Crick and Brenner that ribosomal RNAs were not messenger RNAs after all. Therefore, two nagging key questions remained: (1) What are the messenger RNAs? and (2) Where are they located? So far, three kinds of RNA were known, two ribosomal RNAs and the small transfer RNAs. Since no other RNA was seen, biochemists concluded that messenger RNA must be unstable. Where was it?

It was not until 1958 that these questions began to be answered. The clue that messenger RNA was *not* ribosomal RNA and that it *was* unstable came from an experiment carried out at the Pasteur Institute in Paris by Arthur Pardee, François Jacob (Fig. 10–1), and Jaques Monod (Fig. 10–2). It became known as the PaJaMo experiment or, more colloquially, as the Pajama experiment. In this experiment a gene for the production of an enzyme was transmitted during an *E. coli* mating from a donor strain to a recipient strain that did not possess this gene. The formation of the enzyme was then followed after entry of the gene into the recipient cells. According to Crick's model, it was expected that after entry, the gene would start to produce its ribosomes, that these would accumulate, and that as more and more ribosomes came into operation, enzyme synthesis would steadily accelerate. Instead, what was found was that enzyme synthesis started immediately after entry of the gene at maximal rate. This result was inconsistent with the idea that ribosomal RNA was the messenger RNA.

The conclusion was reinforced by an experiment, carried out later by Pardee with his student, Monica Riley, which showed that not only was the enzyme produced without delay, but enzyme production ceased immediately after the gene was destroyed. They achieved this by incorporating radioactive phosphorus into the DNA template. The decay of the radioactive phosphorus causes breakdown of DNA and destroys the gene. Ribosomes were shown to remain intact under these conditions, and yet enzyme synthesis stopped. This result showed that the presence of the gene was required for continued enzyme synthesis to go on. The result also showed that messenger RNA, which carried the coded information for enzyme synthesis from the gene to the ribosomes, was unstable and had to be continuously produced by the gene.

The enzyme used in the PaJaMo experiment was beta-galactosidase, which catalyzes the breakdown of lactose to glucose and galactose. Lederberg had discovered an easy method for measuring the activity of this enzyme. The enzyme is only produced when its substrate lactose, or a substance structurally related to lactose, is present. It was therefore called an adaptive enzyme. This enzyme was of special interest to Monod who had studied the nature of adaptive enzyme formation for many years. He had begun his studies in the early 1940s at the Pasteur Institute under the tutelage of André Lwoff, an extraordinarily

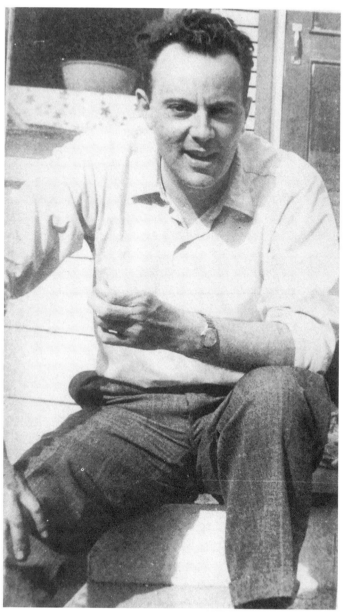

FIGURE 10–1. François Jacob at the Cold Spring Harbor Symposium in 1953. [Courtesy of Cold Spring Harbor Laboratory Library Archives.]

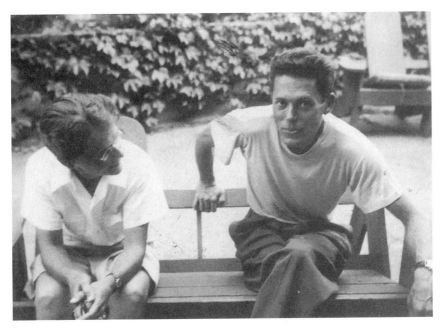

FIGURE 10–2. A youthful Jaques Monod in discussion with Barbara McClintock at the 1947 Cold Spring Harbor Symposium. [Courtesy of Cold Spring Harbor Laboratory Library Archives.]

gifted and original microbiologist (Fig. 10–3). This was during World War II and Monod had just been demobilized from the French army. He carried out his experiments and, at the same time, was active in the French resistance. After the war, he and Lwoff attended a Cold Spring Harbor Symposium and became acquainted with Luria, Delbrück and the rest of the phage group. In the late 1940s and early 1950s several outstanding young American scientists joined Monod at the Pasteur Institute. His laboratory became a Mecca for the study of a new development in molecular genetics, the control of enzyme formation. Much of the attraction of the Paris laboratory was due to the personality of Monod. He was a man of medium height and energetic appearance with a multifaceted range of interests. He was blessed with both great charisma and an incisive power of analysis. Besides being an enthusiastic scientist he was an accomplished cellist and an ardent rock climber, the latter in spite of a greatly weakened leg as a result of childhood polio.

Monod's work was concerned with the genetic control of enzyme formation. Since all enzymes known were proteins, Monod expected that the outcome of his studies would lead eventually to an understanding of how the activity of genes is controlled for determining the structure of proteins. As we see in Chapter 13, the results obtained from the PaJaMo experiment fulfilled these

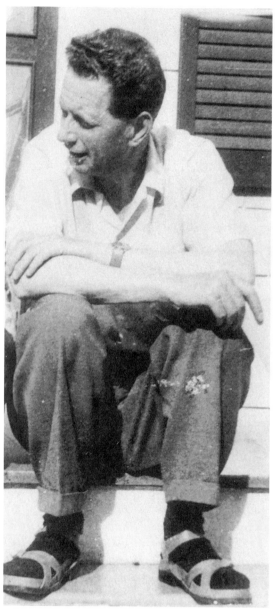

Figure 10–3. André Lwoff at Cold Spring Harbor in 1953. [Courtesy of Cold Spring Harbor Laboratory Library Archives.]

expectations. In the present chapter, we see that they were instrumental in elucidating messenger RNA.

The technical know-how for carrying out the PaJaMo experiment had been created by Jacob and his collaborator, Elie Wollman. They had been studying the mating process of E. coli, discovered by Lederberg in 1946, in which genes are transferred from a donor (male) strain to a recipient (female) strain. In Lederberg's experiments, the frequency of transfer had been quite low, with only 1 in 10,000 male bacteria transferring its genes. Later, in the early 1950s, donor strains were discovered by Luca Cavalli-Sforza in Italy and William Hayes in England that transferred their genes with a very high frequency, with every male bacterium transferring its genes. These strains were called Hfr, which stands for high frequency of recombination. Jacob and Wollman used the Hfr strains isolated by Hayes, called HfrH, in their experiments. The picture that emerged from their studies showed that E. coli contains a single circular chromosome. The ability to act as a donor of genes is due to the presence of a separate small genetic element that could replicate autonomously in the cytoplasm. Lederberg had named this kind of genetic element a plasmid. The plasmid that promoted gene transfer was called a sex factor or an F factor, F standing for fertility. This element itself is transmitted with high frequency during matings. The donor strains that Lederberg had used in 1946 were called F^+, whereas the recipient strains, which did not harbor an F factor, were called F^-. In F^+ strains, F replicates most of the time autonomously but occasionally is integrated into the chromosome. Chromosomal gene transfer is due to these rarely integrated F factors. In Hfr strains, the F factor is permanently integrated at one site of the chromosome. During matings, the circular chromosome breaks at that site and the linear chromosome is transferred to recipient bacteria. Jacob and Wollman had discovered an ingenious method for interrupting matings by treating the mating cultures in a Waring blender, which broke the mating pairs apart. They called this coitus interruptus. This permitted them to time the entrance of genes into the recipient strains. It took 90 minutes at 37°C to transfer the whole chromosome. In the PaJaMo experiment, with the HfrH strain used, the gene for beta-galactosidase synthesis, called lac z^+, began to enter the Lac$^-$ recipient cells after 5 minutes of mating (see Fig. 10–4). Starting from that time, the formation of the enzyme could be measured in the mating mixture.

Jacob is dark-haired, tall, and lanky. He is the intuitive type of scientist with a great deal of imagination. He is an excellent writer. His recent autobiography, La Statue Intérieure, was a bestseller in France. He had studied medicine and planned to become a surgeon, but World War II interrupted his studies. He joined De Gaulle's Free French forces and spent most of the war as a medic in Africa. Having been seriously wounded after his return to France toward the end of the war, he gave up his plans to become a practicing physician. He be-

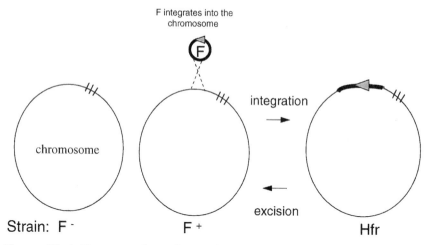

FIGURE 10–4. Formation of an Hfr strain by the integration of an F plasmid into the chromosome. The F plasmid is drawn in a heavy line, with the arrow indicating the origin and direction of transfer. The Hfr strain shown here is called HfrH, named after William Hayes. The three bars represent three lactose genes, *lac* i$^+$, *lac* z$^+$ and *lac* y$^+$ (see Chapter 13), which are transferred to the F$^-$ recipient 5 minutes after initiation of mating.

came attracted to biological research and, after exploring several avenues, ended up, like Monod before him, discussing his future plans with Lwoff. The latter encouraged him to join his department at the Pasteur Institute and Jacob began, together with Wollman, who was an experienced microbiologist, to study the mechanism of gene transfer during *E. coli* matings. He also began to study a bacteriophage, called lambda, which was of special interest to Lwoff.

This phage or bacterial virus, after it infected an *E. coli* cell, had two possible courses of action. It could either multiply and destroy its host or it could join the chromosome and become part of it, living quietly with the other genes. The bacteriophages studied previously by Luria and Delbrück had only the former course open to them. Lwoff referred to lambda as a lysogenic phage because certain agents, such as ultraviolet light, could induce lambda to leave its site in the chromosome and replicate in the cytoplasm, eventually lysing the *E. coli* cell.

It was the study of induction that drew Jacob and Monod together because they saw a parallelism between the induction of quiescent bacteriophages and the induction by lactose, as Monod now called the adaptive process, to produce beta galactosidase. In the beginning they thought that it was only the word induction that they had in common, but as time progressed they realized that there were striking similarities between the induction of bacteriophage lambda and the induction of the enzyme beta-galactosidase. In either case "induction" was a change in the rate of a cellular process involving protein synthesis in response to an environmental agent.

Pardee, the third participant of the PaJaMo experiment had come from the University of California in Berkeley to Paris in the fall of 1957 to work for a year with Monod. He was a brilliant biochemist with a flair for carrying out incisive experiments. In the mid-1950s he showed that the synthesis of beta-galactosidase stopped within minutes when the synthesis of RNA was interrupted. He concluded that continuous synthesis of RNA was essential for protein formation. After his arrival in Paris, Monod proposed to him to carry out an Hfr Lac$^+$ x F$^-$Lac$^-$ mating experiment to get acquainted with the mating system and to be sure that once the females acquired the gene they made the enzyme, and that its appearance could be timed and measured. This is when the PaJaMo experiment was born.

The Pasteur group postulated, based on the previously mentioned outcomes of the PaJaMo experiment and the experiment of Pardee and Riley, that the enzyme was formed on a preformed template, either the DNA itself or more likely an unstable messenger RNA. This RNA would be a copy of the gene and would break down after serving as a template for a few enzyme molecules. This scheme stood in marked contrast to Crick's idea that messenger RNA was a stable RNA associated permanently with a ribosome.

With the new understanding that came from Paris, the nature of the messenger RNA was revealed in Cambridge on Good Friday of 1960. A number of people, including Crick, Brenner, and Jacob, had gathered in Brenner's lodgings at King's College and were discussing the problem of the missing messenger. Crick was questioning Jacob about the validity of their experimental procedures and could not find any faults. I shall quote the vivid description Crick has given in his book, *What Mad Pursuit*, of the scene that followed:

What the PaJaMo [Pardee, Jacob, Monod] type of experiment showed was that ribosomal RNA could not be the message. All the previous difficulties had prepared us for this idea, but we had not been able to take the necessary next step, which was: Where, then, is the message? At that point Sydney Brenner let out a loud yelp—he had seen the answer. (So had I, for that matter, though nobody else had.) One of the peripheral problems of this confused subject had been a minor species of RNA that occurred in *E. coli* shortly after it had been infected by bacteriophage T4. (*E. coli*, a bacterium that lives in our gut, is much used in the laboratory.) Some years earlier, in 1956, two workers, Elliot Volkin and Lazarus Astrachan at the Oak Ridge Laboratory in Tennessee, had shown that (following phage infection) a new species of RNA was synthesized that had an unusual base composition, since it mirrored the base composition of infecting phage and not that of the *E. coli* host, which happened to be very different. They had at first thought that this might be the precursor of the phage DNA, which the infected cell was compelled to synthesize in large quantities, but further work on their part had shown that this hypothesis was incorrect. Their results had hung in midair, surprising but unexplained.

The problem was then: If the messenger RNA was a different species of RNA from ribosomal RNA, then why had we not seen it? What Sidney had seen was that the Volkin-Astrachan RNA *was* the messenger RNA for the phage-infected cell. Once this key insight had been obtained, the rest followed almost automatically. If there was a separate messenger RNA, then clearly a ribosome did not need to contain the sequence for information. It was just an *inert reading head*. Instead of one ribosome being tied to the synthesis of just one protein, it could travel along message, synthesizing the protein, and then go on to a further messenger RNA, where it would synthesize a different protein. The PaJaMo experiment was easily explained by assuming that the messenger RNA was used only a few times before being destroyed.

Actually, the unstable RNA that occurs following infection with phage T2 was first noticed by Hershey during his studies of this phage and later studied in detail by the biochemists Volkin and Astrachan who were not members of the "phage group."

Further along in his account, Crick sums up his experiences of this exciting Good Friday as follows:

> Just a single wrong assumption (that the ribosomal RNA was the messenger RNA) had completely messed up our thinking, so that it appeared as if we were wandering in a dense fog. I woke up that morning with only a set of confused ideas about the overall control of protein synthesis. When I went to bed all our difficulties had resolved and the shining answers stood clearly before us.

Shortly afterwards, Jacob and Brenner set out for California to carry out an experiment that would definitely establish their new hypothesis. Their idea was to distinguish whether, after phage infection, new RNA was present in new ribosomes made after phage infection, or, whether there were no new ribosomes, just the preexisting ones "for hire" to the new messenger RNA made from phage DNA. They carried out this experiment with Matthew Meselson at Caltech. The latter was an expert on the use of heavy and radioactive isotopes for labeling nucleic acids. Previously he had used those techniques for demonstrating the semiconservative replication of DNA (see page 68). After some initial technical difficulties, Brenner and Jacob obtained the results that they expected and they showed that the newly synthesized RNA was associated with the "old" ribosomes. The results were published in the journal *Nature* in a paper entitled "An Unstable Intermediate Carrying Information from Genes to Ribosomes for Protein Synthesis," by S. Brenner, F. Jacob, and M. Meselson.

During the period of the experiment at Caltech, François Gros, an associate of Monod, went to Watson's laboratory at Harvard to study the effect of an antibiotic that inhibited the formation of bacterial ribosomes. In order to follow the formation of ribosomal RNA he used radioactive uracil, a base present in

RNA but not in DNA. In the course of his experiments he found in a control tube without the antibiotic, a species of unstable RNA that resembled neither ribosomal RNA nor transfer RNA. He and Watson had heard about the results of the experiment at Caltech and they went on to show that their unstable RNA was a messenger RNA, this time produced in the absence of infecting phage. At the time, the existence of messenger RNA was also demonstrated in yeast by two other workers, Ycas and Vincent. Within a few years, the existence of unstable messenger RNA was firmly established and the elucidation of the main steps involved in protein synthesis was completed. Messenger RNA, an RNA copy of DNA, was the first intermediary on the way to making protein, including the protein of bacteriophages. It is universally produced and unstable, at least in bacteria.

At about the same time the enzyme responsible for the synthesis of messenger RNA was discovered in extracts of *E. coli* independently in the laboratories of A. Stevens, J. Hurwitz, and S. Weiss. It was named DNA-dependent RNA polymerase. As expected it was found that the base composition of the RNA produced by it is similar to the base composition of the DNA for which it was produced. This enzyme played a key role in subsequent studies on gene action.

The trail leading to messenger RNA was long and twisted: from the laboratory of Hershey at Cold Spring Harbor, to the laboratory of Volkin and Astrachan in Oak Ridge, to the laboratory of Monod and Jacob in Paris, to Crick and Brenner, the theoreticians in Cambridge, and finally to Meselson's laboratory at Caltech and Watson's laboratory at Harvard. Like the Scarlet Pimpernel, messenger RNA was a master in hiding its identity.

With all the steps between genes and their protein products in place, it now remained to determine the correspondence between the codons in DNA and the amino acids in the coded proteins. To do this, it was necessary to decipher the code. In 1960, it was possible to determine the amino acid sequence in proteins, but not the sequence of bases in DNA, which was not worked out until 1977. If DNA sequencing had been possible in 1960, it would have been an easy matter to decipher the code. As it happened, the code was nevertheless deciphered in the early 1960s, thanks to the ingenuity of two young biochemists.

11

Deciphering the Code

THE deciphering of the genetic code was a crowning achievement in the history of molecular genetics. This discovery made it possible to translate the sequence of bases in the DNA of a gene into the sequence of amino acids in the corresponding protein molecule. The heroes of the story were two young biochemists, Marshall Nirenberg and Heinrich Matthaei. Other main actors were the biochemists Severo Ochoa and Har Gobind Khorana and the geneticist George Streisinger. The experimental work was carried out in the early 1960s.

Nirenberg set up his own laboratory at the National Institutes of Health (NIH) in the fall of 1959. He had received his PhD degree in biochemistry in 1957 at the University of Michigan. After 3 years of postdoctoral work at the NIH he was invited to stay on as an independent investigator. In appearance he was tall, dark-haired. He was reserved, not one to advertise his own work. But underneath the surface, there was an intense spirit. His overall aim was to study the flow of information from DNA to protein. To do this he planned to set up a cell-free system for protein synthesis and to add various kinds of nucleic acids to the system as templates to direct the formation of specific proteins. This was before the discovery of messenger RNA, described in Chapter 10.

Matthaei joined Nirenberg in 1960. He had received his PhD degree in 1956 in plant physiology at the University of Bonn. He did research on plant cells for 4 years in Germany before coming to the United states in 1960 on a NATO postdoctoral research fellowship. While still in Germany he reviewed some papers for a journal on cell-free protein synthesis and became interested in the subject. After arriving in the United States he looked for a suitable laboratory to follow up his interest. He first went to see Lipmann, who had moved from Boston to the Rockefeller Institute in New York City, and then saw several people at the NIH. Among them was Nirenberg whom he met in August 1960. After they had discovered their common interests and aims they decided to join forces and Matthaei started to work in Nirenberg's laboratory on November 1. He was 31, Nirenberg was 33. The chief of the laboratory was Leon Heppel, a well-known and skillful biochemist.

As it happened, Heppel had done some work that became very useful for the experiments of Nirenberg and Matthaei. He had become proficient in preparing artificial RNAs of different defined compositions. To do this, he used an enzyme called polynucleotide phosphorylase that catalyzes the formation of RNA. The enzyme had been discovered in 1956 by Marianne Grunberg-Manago and Severo Ochoa at New York University School of Medicine. In 1959 Ochoa was awarded a Nobel Prize for this discovery. Heppel and Ochoa collaborated on analyzing the RNAs that were synthesized with polynucleotide phosphorylase in test tube experiments. By 1960, Heppel and his associate Maxine Singer had accumulated a library of artificial RNAs.

To study protein synthesis, Nirenberg and Matthaei used an *E. coli* preparation developed in Zamecnik's laboratory that was similar to the rat liver cell–free system that had been in use there for several years. The main constituents of the *E. coli* system were ribosomes, transfer RNAs, ATP, guanosine triphosphate (GTP) and amino acids. Protein synthesis was measured by using radioactive amino acids and determining the incorporation of radioactivity into proteins.

The *E. coli* cell-free preparations showed a certain amount of protein synthesis in the absence of added template RNA. This was presumably due to the presence of normal messenger RNA present in the extract. Nirenberg and Matthaei found that this could be eliminated by treatment with the enzyme ribonuclease (RNAse). Once this was done the system was ready to be tested with artificial template RNAs.

In May of 1961 they began to test RNA polymers from Heppel's library. On May 14 Nirenberg left for a 4-week stay in Berkeley, California, and Matthaei did the tests on his own. On May 22 he had worked his way down to three polymers, poly-U, consisting of a long chain of uridylic acids; poly-A, consisting of a long chain of adenylic acids; and a mixed polymer, poly-AU. For incorporation into protein he used a mixture of 16 radioactive amino acids. He found that he got a very high incorporation into protein with poly-U but not with the other two polymers. Now it was a question of finding out which of the amino acids was incorporated. After a strenuous week of testing, he found that it was only phenylalanine that was incorporated. Polyuridilic acid had prompted the cell-free system to put together a unique protein-like substance, a polypeptide composed entirely of phenylalanine. Matthaei had identified the first codon of the genetic code. Assuming that the code is a three-letter code, UUU codes for the amino acid phenylalanine.

After his return from Berkeley Nirenberg learned of Matthaei's success. They carried out some more experiments to finish the identification of the polyphenylalanine peptide and submitted two papers for publication to the *Proceedings of the National Academy of Sciences* on August 3.

Nirenberg presented a paper at the fifth International Congress of Biochemistry that began in Moscow on August 10, 1961. The room was large but almost empty. The title of his talk was not very informative: "The Dependence of Cell-free Protein Synthesis in *E. coli* Upon Naturally Occurring or Synthetic Template RNA." Although this title gave no hint that he and Matthaei had solved the coding problem, there were three people in the audience who understood the significance of his presentation: Walter Gilbert, who later worked out a method for sequencing DNA, Alfred Tissières, an associate of Watson, who worked on protein synthesis with the cell-free *E. coli* system, and Matthew Meselson, who, together with Jacob and Brenner, had carried out the experiment to demonstrate messenger RNA. Afterwards Meselson went to Crick and told him about Nirenberg's report. Crick was chairman of a symposium and he made arrangements for Nirenberg to repeat his talk to a wider audience at this symposium, which took place at the end of the congress. Nirenberg's talk was the last of this session. It was a tremendous climax.

The method developed by Nirenberg and Matthaei was put to immediate use to decipher other codons. While still in Moscow, Nirenberg was told by Matthaei over the phone that he had found polycytidylic acid to direct the synthesis of a polyproline peptide. This meant that CCC was the codon for the amino acid proline. Soon thereafter Ochoa and his coworkers synthesized many polynucleotides that were mixed, i.e., containing more than one base. Such mixed polynucleotides were also available to Nirenberg from Heppel's collection. With these polynucleotides it was possible to produce different polypeptide chains in the *E. coli* cell-free system. A race ensued between Nirenberg's laboratory and Ochoa's laboratory. Within 2 years, 35 different codons could be distinguished by this method, although the order of the three bases within a codon could not always be determined.

In 1964, at the sixth International Congress of Biochemistry in New York City, Nirenberg and his postdoctoral fellow Philip Leder announced a new method for the deciphering of codons that made it possible to determine the order of the three bases. They found that artificial RNAs consisting of only three nucleotides (triplets) could carry out the first step of protein synthesis. In the *E. coli* cell-free system they could bind to ribosomes and there could combine with a complementary transfer RNA attached to its corresponding amino acid. The triplets behaved like a one-word messenger RNA. It contained one codon. As expected, the identity of the amino acid bound depended on the nucleotides present in the triplet and on their sequence.

To detect the amino acid–transfer RNA compounds that were bound to the triplet on the ribosome, they used the neat trick of passing the incubation mixture through a nitrocellulose filter that retained the ribosomes. All the transfer RNA molecules passed through the filter except the ones specifically bound to the ribosomes by the triplet. They could determine which amino acid was retained by using mixtures of amino acids in which one of the amino acids was radioactive. By testing each amino acid in radioactive form, they could identify the bound amino acid by determining the amount of radioactivity absorbed by the filter.

In a previous experiment carried out jointly by Lipmann and Chapeville at Rockefeller University, von Ehrenstein at Johns Hopkins University, and Weisblum, Ray, and Benzer at Purdue University it had been shown that the binding to a codon in messenger RNA is specified by the transfer RNA itself irrespective of the nature of the amino acid attached to it. They used cysteinyl-tRNA bound to radioactive cysteine. In the *E. coli* cell-free system, the radioactivity was transferred to ribosomes in the presence of poly-UG, which supplied the codon UGU for cysteine. They then converted the bound cysteine chemically to alanine. Poly-UG is known *not* to stimulate the transfer to ribosomes of labeled alanine when bound to alanyl-tRNA. However, the radioactive alanine bound to cysteinyl-tRNA was transferred to ribosomes in the presence of Poly-UG, thus showing that the anticodon site in cysteinyl-tRNA was not affected by the nature of the bound amino acid. In later chemical studies on the structure of cysteinyl-tRNA, the anticodon was identified directly by sequencing this tRNA.

Nirenberg and his colleagues synthesized all 64 trinucleotides (triplets) and tested them for their coding properties. Most of the triplets gave an unambiguous answer in the binding test and 50 of the 64 possible codons could be definitely deciphered. It was now clear that most amino acids were coded by more than one codon. The expression used by people in the field to denote this multiplicity of codons for a single amino acid was to say that the code is degenerate.

A direct way to confirm the genetic code was used by the organic chemist Khorana and his colleagues. They synthesized long RNA molecules with a strictly defined base sequence and used them as templates in the *E. coli* cell-free system. As an example they synthesized an RNA molecule with the alternating sequence UGUGUGUGUG . . . Read as triplets, the message will be UGU–GUG–UGU . . . From this, one would expect a polypeptide with alternating amino acids. In fact, they found a peptide with alternating cysteines and valines, with UGU coding for cysteine and GUG coding for valine.

Between Nirenberg's binding technique and Khorana's skill for synthesizing nucleic acids, by 1965 all the codons for the 20 amino acids were established. This amounted to 61 of the 64 possible codons. Three of the triplets, UAA, UAG, and UGA did not code for amino acids. Later it was shown in genetic experiments with bacteriophages by Crick and Brenner, and also by Alan Garen at Yale University, that these three were termination codons that signaled the end of a polypeptide chain. The conditional lethal amber mutants that were first isolated by Epstein (page 56) were due to base changes that generated a UAG triplet. Later, another kind of conditional lethal mutation was found that generated a UAA triplet. Such mutants were named *ochre* mutants. Since such triplets do not code for an amino acid, mutations resulting in such triplets were called nonsense mutations.

The experiments on deciphering the code described so far have all been carried out in extracts, and there was the possibility that the coding is different in intact cells. The main difficulty in carrying out experiments with whole cells, as pointed out before, was that changes in codons as a result of mutation could not (yet) be detected directly by sequencing. It required great ingenuity to show by genetic mapping methods where exactly in the DNA sequence a mutational change had occurred and thus to identify the codon affected by the mutation. The person who developed methods for doing this was Seymour Benzer, mentioned above as a participant in the experiment designed to localize the cysteinyl-tRNA anticodon.

Benzer, trained as a physicist became interested in molecular genetics in the late 1940s, and left physics to join the Phage Group. His mentor was Max Delbrück. He started to work with the bacteriophage T4 and soon discovered a system that permitted him to carry out mapping experiments with a very high degree of resolution. This system is based on the ability of T4 to grow in both *E. coli* B and *E. coli* K12 as hosts. Mutants can be isolated that can grow in *E. coli* B, but not in *E. coli* K12. All these mutants were mapped in a small region of the T4 genome, called the rII region. By infecting *E. coli* B with two such mutants and collecting the resulting phage lysate, one can detect rare recombinants between the two mutants by infecting *E. coli* K12 and plating the infected bacteria on agar petri plates. Recombinant normal phages give rise to clearings on the "lawn" of bacteria on the plates, called plaques. Each plaque is the area of lysis resulting from the growth of a single normal phage in an infected bacterium.

Using this approach Benzer constructed a very detailed map of the rII region. He mapped 350 different sites within this region at which mutations occurred. This number approaches the number of base pairs contained in the DNA of this region. Benzer then asked if the rII region consisted of more than one gene, the gene being defined as the functional unit that enables the phage to grow in *E. coli* K12. To test for this possibility, he infected K12 with two different rII mutants. If the mutations are in different genes, the two mutants should collaborate with each other to grow and lyse the host cells. If they are located within the same gene, they will not collaborate and will not grow. If they do grow, most of the phages in the lysate are still rII mutants. In testing many mutants pairwise, he found that there are two genes in the rII region, which he named A and B. Each gene contains many mutational sites and many sites for recombination. Benzer invented a new terminology: the functional units ordinarily called genes, he named cistrons, based on a test he used, called the cis/trans test. The units for mutation he named mutons and the units for recombination he named recons. The latter two are defined as the smallest region of DNA in which a mutation or a recombination can occur. Presumably, this is a single base pair. The term cistron has been widely accepted and is in common usage.

Benzer was somewhat of a practical joker. As an example, when he delivered a Harvey Lecture in 1960 (at which I was present) he had the genetic map of the rII region with all the mutations on a long scroll of paper that was wound up on two wooden poles. At the beginning of the lecture he asked two dignitaries of the Harvey Society who were sitting in the front row to come up on the stage and to hold up the unrolled map while he proceeded with his talk, referring occasionally to the scroll held up behind him by the two bearers. This went on for a while, until finally they became noticeably restless and somebody in the audience raised his hand and called Benzer's attention to the weakening scroll bearers, at which point Benzer relieved them.

Benzer's system was used by Crick and Brenner to demonstrate that the genetic code was indeed a triplet code. They did this by using an acridine dye as a mutagen that they had proposed to produce deletions or insertions of single base pairs. This was later shown to be correct. With a triplet code such mutations would shift the reading of the code out of frame and they were therefore called frameshift mutants. The mutants that Crick and Brenner studied were in the B cistron of the rII region. The idea behind the experiment was as follows: If one had a single deletion of the first base of a triplet codon, the phage would behave as a mutant. If one added a deletion of the second position in the same or a nearby codon, the phage would still behave as a mutant. However, if one added to the double mutant a deletion of the third position of the codon, the original reading frame would be restored and the resulting triple mutant would behave as a normally functioning phage. Crick and Brenner with their assistant Leslie Barnett carried out appropriate experiments to test this scheme and they found that the triple mutant behaved normally, as expected on the basis of a triplet code. Crick, in his book, *What Mad Pursuit* described the scoring of the crucial experiment, as follows: "Carefully we double-checked the numbers on the petri dishes to make sure we had looked at the correct plate. I looked across at Leslie. 'Do you realize,' I said, 'that you and I are the only people in the world who *know* it's a triplet code?' "

The experiments of Crick and Brenner confirmed that the code is a triplet code, but they did not confirm the code itself. An experiment that did this was carried out by George Streisinger and his colleagues on the enzyme lysozyme of bacteriophage T4. In the normal enzyme, a segment of the protein has the following amino acid sequence: lysine–serine–proline–serine–leucine–asparagine–alanine–alanine–lysine. Streisinger and his coworkers isolated a double frameshift mutant in which the corresponding sequence is lysine–valine–histidine–histidine–leucine–methionine–alanine–alanine–lysine. The changed sequence as the result of the two mutations is underlined. This is the expected change if the first mutation is a deletion of an A in the first serine codon, resulting in a shift of the reading frame, and the second mutation is an insertion of a G in the first alanine, resulting in restoration of the original reading frame. This is strong support for the validity of the code established by Nirenberg because the two mutations alter not only the two amino acids directly affected, but also the amino acids lying between them, as expected from the frame shift in the reading of the codon triplets (see Fig. 11–1).

In his original theoretical considerations of the genetic code, Crick assumed that the code is universal—the same in all organisms. This seems to be largely the case. It was shown that in mutations with base substitutions in three different organisms the change of a single amino acid in the mutant protein could have been caused by the alteration of a single base in the known codon for this amino acid. This was demonstrated for human hemoglobin in 36 mutants, the protein for tobacco mosaic virus in 40 mutants, and the enzyme tryptophan synthetase of *E. coli* in 26 mutants. The total agreement between codon assignment of the normal and mutant amino acids and a single base change in the mutants make it likely that the code is the same in the three organisms. After DNA sequencing became available in 1977, it was established with certainty that the code was, for the most part, universal. The coding mechanism has been preserved during the evolution of living organisms. Presumably, changes in the code would have been lethal.

A concept related to the genetic code that was tested by Benzer's method at the same time as the experiments described above is the sequence hypothesis, which states that the amino acid sequence of a protein is specified by the nucleotide sequence of the gene determining that protein. Brenner, together with three associates, showed that lengths of the protein fragments obtained from different chain-terminating mutants of one of the proteins of T4 agreed with the position of the corresponding mutations in the gene for this protein, as determined by Benzer's mapping procedure. Thus, they established the colinearity of the gene with the protein chain. Similar evidence for colinearity was

WILD TYPE

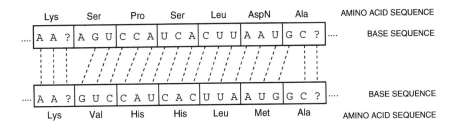

FIGURE 11–1. The altered codons generated in the double frame shift mutant. The deletion of the fourth A causes a change in the codon reading frame, which is restored to the normal frame by the insertion of G 15 base pairs downstream from the deleted A.

obtained at the same time by Charles Yanofsky and his coworkers at Stanford University for the enzyme tryptophan synthetase of *E. coli*. Later, the colinearity was confirmed in both cases by direct sequencing of the mutant genes.

In the history of gene action, the deciphering of the genetic code, as well as the demonstration of colinearity between genes and proteins, are major milestones. They are at the end of a long chain of investigations that started in 1945 with Beadle's statement of the one gene–one enzyme hypothesis. A solid biochemical basis was created for what in 1945 was only a bold hypothesis.

IV

REGULATION OF
GENE ACTION

I N the mid-1950s a development occurred that set a new course for the history of gene action. Until then, gene action was considered to be a process consisting of a linear series of reactions from DNA to protein. Nothing was known about the regulation of this process. Now, studies on the regulation of metabolic pathways were carried out that eventually led to the recognition of genes whose only function was the regulation of the action of other genes. This added a new dimension to the then current concept of gene action. It was no longer confined to a linear process but became part of a circuit that could be turned on or off. Two kinds of genes had to be recognized: structural genes that determine the configuration of enzymes and other cellular proteins, and regulatory genes whose products control the rate of synthesis of proteins encoded by structural genes.

The studies that led to the recognition of regulatory genes were of two kinds. There were the previously mentioned studies on the formation of adaptive enzymes in bacteria that are produced only in response to a nutrient added to the growth medium. The genetic control of this response was studied mainly by Monod in the case of the enzyme beta-galactosidase that is formed in response to the addition of the sugar lactose. The second kind of investigation was concerned with the control of biosynthetic pathways that lead to the formation of the building blocks of macromolecules: amino acids for proteins, and purines and pyrimidines for nucleic acids. It was discovered that each of these building blocks exerted a feedback control over its own formation. When a building block such as an amino acid was added as a nutrient in the growth medium, its synthesis inside the cells was inhibited. This was due to the inhibition of the formation of all the enzymes of the biosynthetic pathway and the inhibition of the activity of the first enzyme.

In 1960, the results of all these studies led to the formulation of a model called the Operon Model that gave a complete picture of gene action and its regulation. It showed how the products of regulatory genes controlled the activity of structural genes. Although this model was based on studies with *E. coli,* it was sufficiently general and flexible to be applicable to work with other organisms. It became a guide for all subsequent studies on gene action.

12

Feedback Control of
Biosynthetic Pathways

FOLLOWING the elucidation of most biosynthetic pathways in the 1940s it became of interest to see how these pathways are controlled. A priori it seemed reasonable to suppose that if an end product of a biosynthetic pathway, such as an amino acid, a purine, or a pyrimidine were supplied in the medium of a growing microorganism such as *E. coli*, it would no longer be necessary for the organism to synthesize this end product. One might expect to find feedback mechanisms that inhibited the formation of the end product. From two kinds of observations it was surmised that such feedback mechanisms actually existed. It was found that in mutants with a block in a biosynthetic pathway (auxotrophs), the substrate for the blocked reaction accumulated and was excreted in the culture medium, *but only at the end of growth,* when the end product of the pathway, which had been supplied as a nutrient, was exhausted. The end product, thus, interfered with its own biosynthesis. The second indication of feedback regulation came from studies on biosynthesis using the technique of isotope dilution. It was found that when *E. coli* was grown with radioactively labeled glucose as a carbon source and an unlabeled amino acid, for example arginine, was added to the growth medium, the subsequently synthesized protein contained only unlabeled arginine.

The indirect evidence from these physiological experiments was substantiated by the direct demonstration of two kinds of mechanisms of feedback control, inhibition by the end product of the formation of the enzymes of a pathway, and inhibition by the end product of the activity of the first enzyme of a pathway.

Feedback inhibition of enzyme formation was first demonstrated in 1953 for methionine synthetase in J. Monod's laboratory at the Pasteur Institute in Paris and in D.D. Woods' laboratory at Oxford University. At the same time it was shown in Monod's laboratory that added tryptophan inhibited the formation of tryptophan synthetase. Both of these enzymes are the last enzymes of the pathway. That feedback inhibition extended to earlier enzymes of a pathway was demonstrated in 1957 in A. Pardee's laboratory at Berkeley for three enzymes of pyrimidine biosynthesis and by Henry Vogel at Yale University and, independently, by myself, for two enzymes of arginine biosynthesis. Vogel, a former colleague from the Davis Laboratory, had demonstrated inhibition of the enzyme acetylornithinase (Fig. 12–1, step E) and I had demonstrated inhibition of the enzyme ornithine transcarbamylase (OTCase) (Fig. 12–1, step F). In his publication in 1957, Vogel coined the term *enzyme repression* to describe this type of feedback control. He named the substance inhibiting enzyme synthesis a *represser* (later the spelling was changed to *repressor*). These terms were generally accepted and have remained in use. During the following years end product repression was demonstrated for most biosynthetic pathways in *E. coli* and in other bacteria, and was found to affect the formation of all of the enzymes in most of the pathways.

My involvement with regulation of arginine biosynthesis began in 1955. At that time I wanted to study how genes control the rate of enzyme synthesis, extending my previous studies that had demonstrated the genetic control of the structure of an enzyme. I therefore looked for mutants in which the *rate* of enzyme synthesis was altered. To do this I screened for conditional cold-sensitive mutants, starting from a completely blocked arginine auxotroph that did not produce OTCase at any temperature (Fig. 12–1, step F). I obtained such mutants that grew at 37°C without arginine, but required arginine for growth at 25°C. This enzyme was easy to measure in extracts. As expected, OTCase was produced after growth at 37°C but not after growth at 25°C. At 25°C, the conditional mutant had to be grown with arginine, but at 37°C it grew in minimal medium without arginine. A surprise came when, as a control, I grew the cells at 37°C with arginine: no OTCase was produced. Subsequently, inhibition of OTCase formation was found in the normal strain as well, both at 37°C and at 25°C. In this roundabout way I had discovered that repression of OTCase is a general phenomenon that had nothing to do with the cold-sensitive mutations.

The second kind of feedback control, inhibition of the activity of the first enzyme of a biosynthetic pathway was first discovered in 1956 in isoleucine biosynthesis of *E. coli* by E. Umbarger, and in pyrimidine biosynthesis of *E. coli* in the same year by R.A. Yates and A. Pardee. In subsequent years, as in the

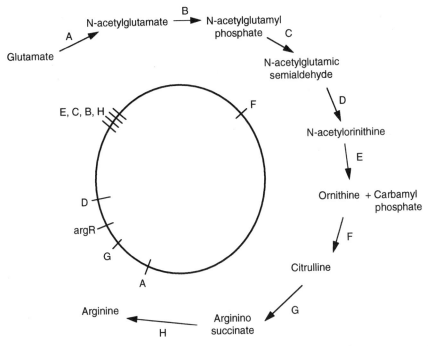

FIGURE 12–1. The enzymatic steps in the biosynthesis of arginine. The map position of the genes controlling these steps is shown in the circular map of the *E-coli* chromosome. The regulatory gene, *argR*, is also shown.

case of enzyme repression, this mechanism was demonstrated in many other biosynthetic pathways. The fact that in all cases it was the first enzyme of a pathway that was inhibited made sense, because this prevents the formation of unnecessary intermediates in the pathways.

Besides the physiological significance of feedback inhibition, the effect poses an interesting question in the biochemistry of enzymes. In most cases, an inhibitor of enzyme activity is structurally related to the substrate. It competes with the substrate for the active site of the enzyme. This is not the case for feedback inhibition. For example, the structure of arginine is quite different from the structure of glutamic acid (Fig. 12–1). In the jargon of biochemistry, structurally related inhibitors are said to be isosteric analogs of the substrate. Monod introduced the term allosteric for inhibitors that are unrelated to the substrate, as is the case for end product inhibition. In structural terms this means that the inhibitor acts at a site on the enzyme molecule that is different from the active site for the substrate. The concept of allostery became very important in regulation of metabolic processes and, as is discussed later, in Chapters 14 and 15, plays a major role in the control of enzyme formation.

After discovering that added arginine repressed enzyme synthesis, I became interested in the question of whether or not internally produced arginine could produce the same effect. I made an observation that suggested that this was indeed the case. This came about when I found an unexpected result in a study of the rate (kinetics) of OTCase formation following the removal of arginine from a growing culture of *E. coli*. At that time kinetics of enzyme formation had been studied by Monod for the formation of beta-galactosidase after addition of lactose. He found that the enzyme was produced at a constant rate for several hours. In the case of OTCase there was an initial burst of enzyme synthesis for about 20 minutes followed by a sharp decrease in the rate. To explain this unexpected result I postulated that during the initial burst arginine would be made rapidly in the cells and the accumulated arginine would inhibit further OTCase synthesis. The problem was to design an experiment that would test this explanation.

At that time in 1956, I was joined by a visiting investigator from Italy, Luigi Gorini. He had been very active in the resistance against the Germans in Italy during World War II. After the war, he did biochemical research in Paris for several years prior to coming to New York. Of medium stature, with blue eyes and brown hair, his appearance was characteristic of some Northern Italians. He was very enthusiastic about his work and full of original ideas. He was a very amusing speaker and kept the constant attention of his audience by thought-provoking pronouncements delivered in his idiosyncratic brand of English. To me he was a stimulating colleague and we had a fruitful collaboration for 3 years. After that he moved to Harvard Medical School where he continued studies on the regulation of arginine biosynthesis, as is described later in this chapter and in Chapter 14. Later he made important contributions to the elucidation of ribosome function in protein synthesis.

In looking for a way to test the idea that the arrest of OTCase synthesis was due to accumulated arginine, we had to find conditions under which arginine would not accumulate. We learned that such conditions could be obtained by growing mutant bacteria requiring arginine for growth in an ingenious device called a chemostat. In this device the internal concentration of arginine could be reduced to a level that made arginine the limiting factor for protein synthesis and, therefore, for growth.

The chemostat had been invented by the eminent Hungarian physicist Leo Szilard, who had previously been instrumental in designing the atomic bomb (Fig. 12–2). He and Enrico Fermi had constructed the first successful atomic pile at the University of Chicago. After Hiroshima and Nagasaki, Szilard became disillusioned with physics and the potentially destructive influence it had on society so he switched to biology. Together with Aaron Novick, a physical chemist whom he had met during the development of the atomic bomb at Los Alamos, he set up a laboratory for the (more peaceful) study of bacterial genet-

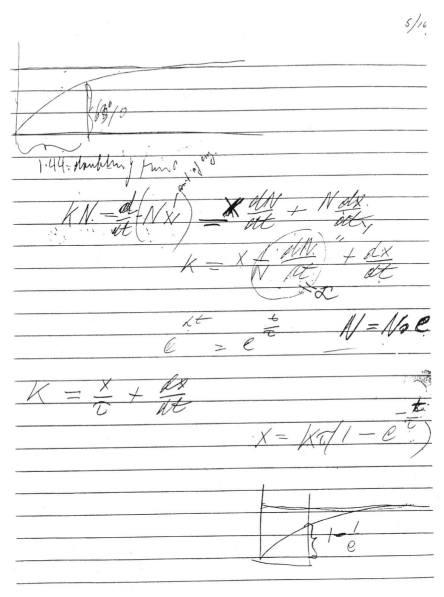

FIGURE 12–2. In 1956, during a discussion with the author, Leo Szilard wrote on a sheet of paper the equations for enzyme formation in chemostat experiments.

ics and physiology at the University of Chicago. It was there that he invented the chemostat. (Monod, independently, invented a similar device called a bactogen.)

Szilard was an extraordinary man. He was quite short and pudgy, the latter characteristic not being helped by his love of rich food. He took a great interest in all the advances that were made in molecular genetics and he, like a gadfly, spent most of his time visiting other scientists who were working in the field, discussing their work with them and often giving them invaluable advice. He would appear suddenly, carry out a pertinent discussion and, after having satisfied his intentions, disappear just as abruptly. Although he was nominally a professor at the University of Chicago, nobody was ever sure of his whereabouts. I met him first in 1951 and had frequent discussions with him over the next 10 years. When I studied the temperature-sensitive mutant in Davis' laboratory, he made some excellent suggestions for experiments that demonstrated the point I wanted to prove. Later, when Luigi and I faced the problem of finding the proper conditions of testing for the control of enzyme production by internally produced arginine, it was Szilard and Novick who suggested the use of the chemostat during a conversation we had in New York.

Our experiments with the chemostat showed that under conditions of arginine-limited growth, OTCase was produced at a very high and constant rate, as expected from "Monod kinetics." The enzyme was produced 100 times as fast as under normal conditions of growth without added arginine. We concluded that the bacteria have a very high capacity for making OTCase, but that the formation of the enzyme is throttled down to a low level by internally produced arginine. Later it was shown that this kind of regulation was found for all the enzymes of arginine biosynthesis. Moreover, it was found in other biosynthetic pathways that were studied at the time. It was recognized as a general principle that feedback control of enzyme formation maintains enzymes at a low level, sufficient for normal growth, but that there is lots of reserve capacity for enzyme synthesis when emergency conditions arise that require a rapid synthesis of the end product of a metabolic pathway.

It seemed unlikely that the end product by itself could bring about the inhibition of a diverse group of enzymes. We therefore expected that there must be another substance that worked in conjunction with the end product to bring about this effect. One possibility of finding this substance was to look for mutants that were no longer repressible by the end product.

In the case of several amino acids there were chemical analogs known that inhibit growth by competing with the amino acid in protein synthesis. One could look for mutants that were resistant to the growth-inhibitory effects of such analogs. This could be explained by the loss of repression that would result in overproduction of the competing amino acid.

In the case of arginine such an analog is canavanine, a naturally occurring substance produced by canava beans. Inhibition of growth by canavanine can be overcome by the addition of arginine.

I started to isolate canavanine-resistant mutants in 1957 together with my associates James Schwartz and Eric Simon. At that time we used a strain of *E. coli*, called *E. coli* W. All the mutants we isolated were still repressible, like the parent strain. Their resistance was shown later to be because of a defect in the uptake mechanism (permease) for arginine, which also reduced the uptake of canavanine. During the summer of 1959 while I was a visitor in Jacob's laboratory at the Pasteur Institute in Paris, I again looked for canavanine-resistant mutants, this time in *E. coli* K12. I used OTCase formation as an indicator of repressibility. The first mutants I isolated were derepressed for OTCase. Later they were shown to be derepressed also for other enzymes of the arginine pathway. Similar derepressed mutants were isolated in Gorini's laboratory in Boston, using another method of selection. In mapping experiments, all the mutations were found at the same site in the chromosome, suggesting that they affected the same gene. The gene was named ArgR, the R standing for regulator. The product of the ArgR gene presumably was able to regulate, in conjunction with arginine, the production of all the enzymes of the arginine pathway. The product of ArgR was named the arginine repressor. Arginine itself was named the corepressor.

Shortly afterwards the genes for the eight enzymes of arginine biosynthesis were mapped in our laboratory and in Gorini's laboratory. We used the interrupted mapping technique of Jacob and Wollman described in Chapter 10. We found that the genes were located in several sites in the circular chromosome, with none of them overlapping the site of ArgR. Yet they were all controlled by the product of the ArgR gene.

The results of the mapping experiments were surprising given that for several other pathways such as tryptophan biosynthesis and histidine biosynthesis, the genes were found to be next to each other. In fact, for these pathways, the order of the genes in the chromosome was found to be the same as the sequence of the reactions in the pathway. M. Demerec and P.E. Hartman, in reviewing the experiments with tryptophan and histidine biosynthesis carried out at Cold Spring Harbor, referred to a cluster of genes for one pathway as a complex locus. Locus designates the region in the chromosome occupied by a gene.

The astonishing arrangement of gene clusters suggested that there is some kind of functional unity for a cluster. This idea was strengthened by the finding of Bruce Ames and Barbara Garry that the level of all the enzymes in the histidine pathway changed to the same extent with different degrees of repression by histidine. Such coordinate repression was not found for the enzymes of arginine biosynthesis where the genes are scattered. These findings foreshadowed the emergence of operons as units of gene expression that are described in Chapter 14.

Regulatory genes, analogous to ArgR, were also found for other pathways. For example, in 1959 Georges Cohen and François Jacob isolated mutants of *E. coli* that were resistant to growth inhibition by 5-methyl tryptophan, an analog of tryptophan. These mutants were derepressed for all the enzymes of the tryptophan pathway. The mutations occurred within the same gene, which was named TrpR. The TrpR gene is not within the cluster of the genes for trypto-phan biosynthesis.

An interesting variation in the regulation of arginine biosynthesis was discovered by Gorini. He found that in *E. coli* B, in contrast to *E. coli* K12, addition of arginine during growth caused an increase in enzyme levels, rather than the decrease seen in *E. coli* K12. Gorini studied this puzzling difference and found that it was due to a difference in the ArgR genes of the two strains. He died in 1976 and I continued to study this problem. In 1986, when sequencing techniques were available, Dongbin Lim, a graduate student and I found that there was a single amino acid difference because of a single nucleotide change between ArgR of *E. coli* B and ArgR of *E. coli* K12, but it was not until 1992 that we discovered how this single amino acid change could bring about the altered response to the addition of arginine.

The main questions that arose from the studies on feedback regulation of enzyme synthesis were: (*1*) What is the chemical nature of the repressor? Is it a protein or a nucleic acid? (*2*) Where is the site of action of the repressor in the synthesis of biosynthetic enzymes? Is it on the DNA or on the messenger RNA?

In regard to the first question, a clue was provided by the requirement of arginine to act as a corepressor. Arginine (and other amino acids) is required for feedback inhibition of the first enzyme of the pathway, and there it has been shown that it interacts with the enzyme to produce its allosteric effect. In analogy with this finding, it seemed likely that the site of action of arginine was a protein produced by ArgR. However, a definite answer was not obtained until about 10 years later when the products of regulatory genes began to be isolated and were shown to be proteins.

In regard to the second question, it was answered within 2 years by the experiments of Monod and his colleagues at the Pasteur Institute, as we see in Chapter 13.

13

Adaptive Enzymes

═══════════════════════════

═══════════════════════════

THE history of adaptive enzymes, like the history of repressible enzymes, starts from the recognition of an adaptive physiological process and goes from there to the regulation of metabolic pathways and then to the control of gene action by specialized genetic elements. This chapter discusses how the two separate approaches leading to the control of gene action met in 1958 and resulting in a unified hypothesis.

The phenomenon of enzymatic adaptation has been known for a much longer time than end product repression. It was described around 1900 by several microbiologists including F.A. Went who demonstrated it in *Neurospora*. In the 1930s it was studied extensively by the Finnish microbiologist H. Karström who classified enzymes into two groups, adaptive enzymes that were produced only in the presence of a substrate and constitutive enzymes that were produced under any condition of growth.

Monod became involved in enzymatic adaptation through a study of the kinetics of bacterial growth that he carried out as a student at the University of Paris. He observed that when he used two different carbon sources for growth, there were two separate growth phases but, that this occurred only with some pairs and not with others. For example, glucose and lactose gave a diphasic growth curve. Monod named this type of growth *diauxie*. He showed his data to Lwoff at the Pasteur Institute. In his Nobel Lecture (he received the Nobel

Prize with Jacob and Lwoff in 1965) he describes this meeting as follows: "Lwoff, after considering this strange result of diphasic growth for a moment, said to me 'That could have something to do with enzyme adaptation.' 'Enzyme adaptation? Never heard of it,' I said." In reply, Lwoff gave him a list of references and after studying them he became convinced that Lwoff's intuition had been correct. The phenomenon of diauxie was closely related to enzyme adaptation and he decided to investigate it. As he stated later in his Nobel lecture: "The die was cast. Since that day in December 1940, all my scientific activity has been devoted to the study of this phenomenon."

Monod's interests were in both the biochemistry and the genetics of adaptive enzyme formation. His interest in genetics had been aroused earlier at Caltech, where he stayed together with his friend, Boris Ephrussi. There he became acquainted with the members of the Morgan group. This interest was reinforced later when he attended the Cold Spring Harbor Symposium in 1946.

As mentioned before, Monod concentrated his studies on the adaptive utilization of lactose and especially on the adaptive formation of the enzymes beta-galactosidase that splits lactose into galactose and glucose. Much of his work was carried out in collaboration with Melvin Cohn, a young American immunologist, who had come to his laboratory in 1948. The following crucial characteristics of the lactose system were established by Monod, Cohn, and any other American or French collaborator who happened to be in the laboratory at the time.

1. It was shown that not only lactose, but a number of compounds structurally related to lactose could elicit formation of beta-galactosidase. Some of these galactosides were not split by the enzyme. There were other galactosides that were split, that is, they were substrates for the enzyme but they did not elicit enzyme formation. Because of this separation between utilization as carbon source and stimulus of enzyme formation, Monod replaced the teleological term adaptive enzyme formation with the more neutral term enzyme induction. Substances that elicited enzyme formation were called *inducers*.

2. Monod and coworkers showed that upon addition of an inducer, the enzyme was produced at a constant rate, proportional to the rate of growth of the bacteria. In the absence of added inducer, the enzyme was also produced but at a very slow rate. The function of the inducer was to greatly increase the rate of enzyme formation.

3. By using a radioactive amino acid as tracer, they showed that the enzyme was synthesized de novo from amino acids. There was no turnover in which the enzyme would be formed by the partial breakdown of other proteins present in the cell.

4. It was found that, in addition to beta-galactosidase, there were two other entities whose formation was elicited by inducers. One was a specific transport system that brought beta-galactosides into the cell. Monod coined the term permease to denote such specific transport systems. The gene for the permease was called *lac y*. The other was an enzyme that acetylated beta-galactosides. It was never shown what function, if any such acetylated beta-galactosides have in the metabolism of the cell. The gene for it was called *lac a*. It is located next to *lac y*, but for simplicity's sake it is not shown on any of the diagrams.

5. Many different kinds of mutants were isolated. Some of these affected only one of the three entities of the lactose system others affected all three. The latter were pleiotropic. There were two types of pleitropic mutants: either they did not produce any of the three entities or they produced all three at a high rate without any added inducer. Monod denoted the gene for the pleiotropic behavior as *lac I* (for inducibility). Previously Lederberg had isolated similar pleiotropic mutants and called them constitutive mutants. As mentioned before, Lederberg had developed a method for measuring the activity of the enzyme that greatly facilitated such studies. It consisted of measuring the development of a yellow color that was produced when the enzyme split the colorless galactoside o-nitrophenyl-galactose (ONPG) into o-nitrophenol and galactose. This method is used universally.

Monod had early on formed a hypothesis about enzyme induction. A gene would direct synthesis of an inactive enzyme protein that would then become activated by interaction with an inducer. He based his hypothesis on a theory for the formation of specific antibodies that had been proposed by Pauling in 1940. Pauling's idea was that inactive precursor protein molecules were molded into completed antibodies when they came in contact with an antigen. For example, diphtheria toxin, a good antigen, could elicit the production of a complete antibody that subsequently was able to inactivate the toxin. On the basis of his hypothesis, Monod interpreted constitutive mutants as producers of an internal inducer, that obviated the necessity for adding an inducer. Monod was a strong believer in a unitary hypothesis for the control of enzyme formation. To explain the inhibition of tryptophan synthetase formation and methionine synthetase formation described in Chapter 12, he postulated that in these cases the end product inhibited the inducing action of the internally produced substrate of the enzyme. Thus, he explained the inhibition of tryptophan synthetase formation by saying that tryptophan inhibits the inducing action of indolglycerol phosphate, the substrate of the enzyme, which is produced as an intermediary during tryptophan biosynthesis. In his view, the primary action was the induction of enzyme formation by its substrate and the inhibition of this induction by tryptophan was a secondary effect.

Monod's hypothesis was in conflict with the results of the chemostat experiments that Gorini and I had performed on the formation of OTCase. For these experiments we had used an arginine-requiring mutant that was genetically blocked in the formation of ornithine, the substrate of OTCase. Yet it produced this enzyme at a very high rate during arginine-limited growth. These results ruled out the internal inducer hypothesis, since ornithine was not produced. On the basis of a unitary hypothesis for the control of enzyme formation, one had to assume that adaptive enzyme formation is due to the removal of a normally present repressor and that inducers act by removing the action of repressors. The primary action is repression, and the inducer acts secondarily by removing repression.

In April 1957, I attended the Federation Meetings in Chicago and stayed at the Quadrangle Club where Szilard was also staying. I met him during breakfast and told him about the conclusion I had reached regarding enzyme induction from the results of the chemostat experiments. Szilard was impressed with my hypothesis and said that it could explain some results they had obtained in their own laboratory.

Early in 1958, Szilard presented the alternative unitary hypothesis at a seminar at the Pasteur Institute. At that time, Pardee had just begun to carry out the PaJaMo experiment. The thinking of Monod was still in favor of an internal inducer hypothesis but it appears that Szilard's seminar and the subsequent discussion had a strong influence in convincing him of the validity of the inhibition of repression hypothesis.

As he stated in his Nobel lecture:

> Of course, I had learned, like any schoolboy that two negatives are the equivalent to a positive statement, and Melvin Cohn and I, without taking it too seriously, debated this logical possibility that we called "the theory of the double bluff," recalling the subtle analysis of poker by Edgar Allan Poe.
>
> I see today, however, more clearly than ever, how blind I was in not taking this hypothesis seriously sooner, since several years earlier we had discovered that tryptophan inhibits the synthesis of tryptophan synthetase, the enzyme that produces tryptophan from its precursors; also, the subsequent work of Vogel, Gorini, Maas, and others showed that repression is not due, as we had thought, to an antiinduction effect. I had always hoped that the regulation of "constitutive" and inducible systems would be explained one day by a similar mechanism.

Later in his lecture he said:

> Why not suppose, then, since the existence of repressible systems and their extreme generality were now proven, that induction could be effected by an antirepressor, rather than repression by an antiinducer? this is precisely the thesis that Leo Szilard, while passing through Paris, happened to propose to us during a seminar. We had only recently obtained the first results of the injection (Pajama) experiment, and we were still not sure about its interpretation. I saw that our preliminary observations confirmed Szilard's penetrating intuition, and when he had finished his presentation, my doubts about the theory of the "double bluff" (induction equals removal of repression) had been removed.

The results of the completed PaJaMo experiment did indeed establish the validity of the removal of a repressor model. It should be noted that in mating experiments of this kind the Hfr donor strain contributes only its genes to the resulting zygote, whereas the recipient strain contributes both its genes and its cytoplasm. Actually, two reciprocal matings were carried out. In the first, the donor strain contributed the constitutive i^- gene (producing an internal inducer, according to Monod) and an inactive z^- gene for the enzyme. The recipient strain contained the gene for inducibility i^+ (producing a repressor according to my hypothesis) and a normal gene for the enzyme, z^+. In this mating, no enzyme was produced in the resulting zygotes, unless an external inducer, such as thiomethyl galactoside (TMG) was added. In the reciprocal cross, the donor Hfr strain contributed the z^+ and i^+ genes and the recipient strain contributed the z^- and i^- genes. In this case, enzyme was produced immediately after entry of the z^+ gene into the zygotes. The genetic constitution of the diploid zygotes formed in the two experiments was the same: z^+i^+/z^-i^-. The only difference was who contributed the cytoplasm: the z^+i^+ strain or the z^-i^- strain. In the former case, no enzyme was formed in the presence of the i^+ gene, even after the i^- gene had entered. In the latter case, enzyme was formed in the i^- cytoplasm of the zygotes, but it was only temporary (90 minutes), until the transferred i^+ gene was expressed. The results showed that the gene for inducibility, i^+, was dominant over the gene for constitutivity, i^-. The findings clearly favored the "induction equals removal of repression" hypothesis over Monod's hypothesis of an "internal inducer." Later, the former hypothesis was shown to be correct by carrying out direct biochemical experiments.

E. coli normally carries one copy of each gene—it is haploid. During a mating it becomes diploid for the genes that have entered, but this state is transitory until the entering genes have recombined with the corresponding resident genes. It was therefore desirable to find strains that were permanently diploid for the Lac genes (lac z, lac y, lac a). A method for constructing such strains was developed by Edward Adelberg, a visiting scientist from Yale University. The method was based on the formation of autonomously replicating F plasmids (see Chapter 10) in Hfr strains that had acquired a piece of the bacterial chromosome, as indicated in the diagram below. The F plasmids containing a piece of chromosomal DNA were called F-prime (F'). The strain that Adelberg and Jacob used for their experiments was isolated from an Hfr strain in which the F plasmid was inserted next to the three lactose genes. The F' plasmid they obtained was called F'lac. The F factor was inserted in such a way that the lac genes would be at the end of the chromosome transferred by the resulting Hfr strain (see Fig. 13–1). In this way they could isolate F-lac elements by selecting for Lac+ colonies in the Hfr lac+ x F-lac− matings that were interrupted early, before the end of the chromosome had entered the recipient cells. The early

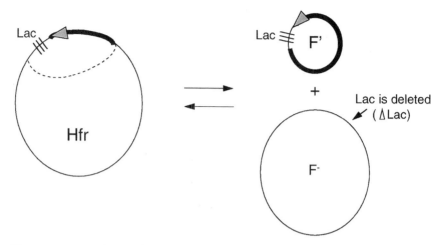

Figure 13–1. Isolation of an F′lac plasmid. In the Hfr strain used, the *lac* genes are located at the terminus of the transferred chromosome. Chromosomal *lac*⁺ recombinants are therefore formed only after about 90 minutes of mating. Any F′lac elements that are present in the Hfr culture are transferred early during the mating. They can be selected by screening for Lac⁺ colonies after early interruption of the mating.

interruption of chromosome transfer prevented the formation of ordinary *Lac*⁺ recombinants.

With the F′*lac* strain they created permanent diploids that carried the normal *lac* genes i⁺, z⁺, y⁺ in the chromosome and the mutant *lac* genes i⁻, z⁻, y⁻ in the F′*lac* plasmid (or vice versa). In these strains the enzyme was produced only after addition of an inducer thus confirming the dominance of the *lac* i⁺ gene over the *lac* i⁻ gene.

Jacob realized that the existence of a specific repressor required that the protein-synthesizing machinery must contain a site at which the repressor acts in order to block protein synthesis. Since the repressor is endowed with specificity, the receptor site is also specific and should therefore be genetically determined. It should be possible to isolate mutants in the receptor site that could no longer respond to the repressor and would be constitutive or deregulated for enzyme synthesis, like *lac* i⁻ mutants. The question was how one could distinguish between *lac* i⁻ mutants and mutants in the receptor site.

Jacob foresaw the answer to this question by thinking about the expected behavior of such mutations in diploid strains. Mutants due to a mutation in the *lac* i gene are recessive (do not express) to normal inducible strains, as we have seen above. Mutations in a receptor site for the repressor would be expected to be dominant (not receptive), because the repressor, produced by the normal *lac i*+ gene, cannot exert its action. Such mutants, even in the presence of a normal *lac i*+ gene, would produce the enzyme in the absence of added inducer.

Jacob proceeded to isolate many constitutive mutants in which both the enzyme and the permease were produced without the addition of an inducer. He used the two characteristics together to detect pleiotrophic mutants. He then introduced an F'*lac* plasmid into them that had normal *lac z*+ and *lac y*+ genes. Most of the resulting diploids became enzyme and permease negative without the inducer, but some of them retained their ability to produce enzyme and permease. The latter were the desired receptor site dominant mutants. Jacob named the receptor site for the repressor an operator (O). The mutations in O were mapped and found to be next to the *lac z* gene and the *lac y* gene.

The study of *lac*O mutants led Jacob to the notion that the genetic material of *E. coli* is organized into genetic units of regulation, which he called operons. An operon consists of one or more genes that are controlled by a single operator. The operator, in turn, is controlled by a repressor. As we see in Chapter 14, Jacob and Monod built a general model of gene action and its regulation on the concept of the operon.

14

The Operon Model

THE culmination of the work on gene action and its regulation occurred in 1961 with the formulation of the Operon Model by Jacob and Monod. This combined all the steps of protein synthesis, so carefully assembled since 1953, with the regulatory mechanisms described in Chapters 12 and 13, in a complete picture. It was a peak in the history of gene action from which one could view the past and obtain a glimpse of the future.

The Operon Model was unveiled at the Cold Spring Harbor Symposium in the Spring of 1961 (Fig. 14–1). Many of the people who provided its building blocks presented papers at the symposium. Bernard Davis gave the opening lecture on "The Teleonomic Significance of Biosynthetic Control Mechanisms." Sydney Brenner and François Gros spoke about their work on messenger RNA. Jerard Hurwitz reported on the DNA-dependent RNA polymerase. Mahlon Hoagland discussed his studies on cell-free protein synthesis. Papers dealing with the regulation of enzyme synthesis were presented by the Arginine Trio, Henry Vogel, Luigi Gorini, and I, by Michael Yarmolinsky, Aron Novick, and Norman Horowitz, among others. Edwin Umbarger talked about his work on feedback inhibition. Present in the audience were Fritz Lipmann, Milislav Demerec, Rollin Hotchkiss, Salvador Luria, Al Hershey, and Jim Watson.

The unveiling of the model was done by Jacob. The diagram of the Operon Model that he presented, shown in Figure 14–1 illustrates the connection be-

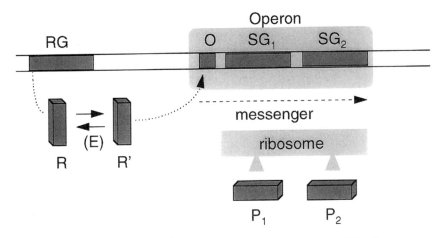

Figure 14–1. The Operon Model. The repressor R is converted to R′ in the presence of an effector E (inducing or repressing metabolite). It acts on the operator O. P_1 and P_2 are the protein products of the two structural genes.

tween regulatory genes (RG) and structural genes (SG). The model is based on the lactose operon, in which there is the regulatory gene *lac i* (RG) that makes a repressor (R), and two structural genes, *lac z* (SG1), that makes the enzyme and, next to it, *lac y* (SG2), a gene that controls the transport of lactose into the cell. (In his diagram he left out the gene for the acetylating enzyme.)

Jacob characterized the features of the Operon Model as follows (parentheses are mine):

1. The primary product of structural genes, or *"messenger RNA,"* which brings structural information from genes to cytoplasmic protein-forming centers, is a short-lived intermediate. Once completed, it is detached from the DNA and associates in the cytoplasm with preexisting, nonspecialized ribosomal particles. The second transcription (translation) takes place on ribosomes, and the messenger is destroyed in the process. Once completed, the polypeptide (protein) folds and is detached from the ribosomal particle, which is set free for a new transcription cycle involving the same or any other specific messenger.

2. The synthesis of messenger RNA is supposed to be a sequential and oriented process which can be initiated only at certain regions, or *operators* (O), on the DNA strands. In many instances, a single operator may control the transcription of several adjacent structural genes. Such a group of genes, whose transcriptive activity is thus coordinated by a single operator, constitutes an *operon*. The operon may therefore be defined as the unit of primary transcription.

3. The genetic material contains determinants functionally distinct from structural genes, called regulator genes. A regulator gene produces a cytoplasmic *repressor*. The repressor formed by a given regulator gene has an affinity toward, and tends to associate reversibly with, a specific operator. This combination

blocks the initiation of transcription of the whole operon controlled by the operator and therefore prevents the synthesis of the proteins governed by the structural genes belonging to the operon.

4. The repressors have the property of reacting with certain small molecules which we shall call effectors. The reactions are specific with respect to both the repressors (R) and the effectors (F) and may be expressed as

$$R + F \leftrightarrow R' + F'$$

In certain systems, called *inducible* (such as the Lactose Operon), only the R form of the repressor can associate with the operator and block the transcription of the operon. The presence of the effector, called inducer, inactivates the repressor and therefore allows transcription to take place. In other systems, called *repressible* (such as the genes of arginine biosynthesis), only the modified repressor (R') is active. (In this case, the effector is called a corepressor.) The transcription of the operon, allowed in the absence of the effector is therefore prevented in its presence.

This model may appear rather complex and abstract. It is, however, precise enough to imply very distinctive predictions by which its validity can be tested. In the course of the discussion that follows we hope to show that, although some details of the mechanisms are speculative, the main outlines of this scheme are not pure assumptions and that, in its major features, it is firmly grounded on experimental evidence. Before discussing the evidence, it may be useful to state clearly these "major features."

a. The first postulate is the distinction between two classes of genes, structural and regulatory, which fulfill different functions in the genetic control of protein synthesis.

b. The second is the postulate that the regulatory mechanisms, in inducible and repressible systems as well as in lysogenic systems (involving bacteriophages), are primarily *negative*, i.e., operate by inhibiting, rather than provoking, specific protein synthesis. (He is referring to his work with phage lambda.)

c. The third is the postulate that *several* linked structural genes may constitute a coordinated unit of transcriptive activity.

d. The fourth is the postulate that the regulatory mechanisms operate at the genetic level, by controlling the rate of synthesis of the messenger.

e. The fifth is the postulate that the primary gene product (messenger) is a short-lived intermediate.

During the remainder of his talk, Jacob described results of experiments that he and Monod had carried out with the lactose system and that led to the formulation of the Operon Model. To begin with, he referred to the work on messenger RNA, which Sidney Brenner had described in a previous talk of the symposium recounting the story of its discovery (see Chapter 10). After that he described the evidence for the repressor and the operator, as shown in the model. This evidence was based mainly on the properties of regulatory mutants in the lactose system and the interaction of these mutants with their normal counterparts. The evidence that he presented for a single messenger RNA that included both structural genes and that was initiated at O was, simply, that mutations in O eliminated the response to the repressor for beta galactoside and permease. He interpreted this to mean that the repressor prevented the synthesis of a common messenger RNA for both structural genes at the operator site.

After Jacob's Cold Spring Harbor talk it became clear that the Operon Model was a general scheme that applied to other cases of gene-controlled protein synthesis, besides the lactose operon. It explained, for example, the puzzling observations that Demerec and Hartman had made at Cold Spring Harbor in the 1950s. As mentioned before, they had found that the genes of the pathway for tryptophan biosynthesis and the genes for histidine biosynthesis were next to each other in the chromosome. This initially mysterious finding could now be explained by saying that the group of genes for each pathway constituted an operon.

Although the Operon Model was clearly a benchmark in the history of molecular genetics, a few of its features had to be modified. At the time of the Cold Spring Harbor Symposium, Jacob and Monod had concluded that the repressor consisted of RNA, based on experiments that showed that repressor was produced in the presence of inhibitors of protein synthesis. However, later it was found that they had misinterpreted the experiments and that the evidence was not conclusive. Moreover, from studies on certain mutant types of the repressor, especially temperature sensitive mutants, gradually the evidence grew stronger that the repressor was a protein. The idea of a protein repressor seemed strange because it was difficult to see how proteins, being so different from nucleic acids, could bind to DNA. It was much simpler to imagine RNA binding to DNA. Nevertheless, these reservations had to be laid to rest in 1966, when the Lac repressor was isolated in pure form by Walter Gilbert and Benno Müller-Hill at Harvard and shown to be a protein.

Gilbert was originally a member of the Physics Department at Harvard, but became fascinated by molecular genetics. He joined Watson's group in 1960 and took part in the experiments of Watson and Gros that demonstrated the existence of unstable messenger RNA. After his successful isolation of the Lac repressor he developed a method for sequencing DNA that is still widely used. He was awarded a Nobel Prize for this work.

Müller-Hill was a German postdoctoral student in Gilbert's laboratory. He has continued his study of the Lac repressor and other repressors until the present. He is now a professor at the University of Cologne. Besides his experimental work, he has devoted himself to investigate and publicize the infamous activities of German biologists during the Nazi period.

A modification of the Operon Model arose in connection with the work on the regulation of arginine biosynthesis. In my talk given during the symposium I described the mutants I had isolated in the biosynthesis of arginine and in the formation of the repressor, ArgR. At the end I presented a general model of how this repressor, by interacting with arginine, the corepressor, inhibits the formation of all the enzymes of arginine biosynthesis. The model, a modification of the Operon Model, is shown in Figure 14–2. I named it a Multiple-Operator Model.

The reason for the modification was that the eight genes for the biosynthesis of arginine were not all next to each other, as postulated in the Operon Model, but four of them were scattered separately over the chromosome. There could thus not be a single messenger RNA for the eight genes. Yet I had found that the formation of all eight enzymes was controlled by the arginine repressor, the product of the regulatory gene ArgR.

In the diagram, the repressor acts at three operator sites. Actually, for arginine biosynthesis there are five separate operator sites, one for a cluster of four structural genes and four for the four single structural genes. In 1964, John Clark and I coined the word *Regulon* to describe a unit of regulation, where a single repressor controls the formation of enzymes of a pathway in which the genes for the separate enzymes are not next to each other. We postulated that the five operator sites had to be very similar to combine with the same repres-

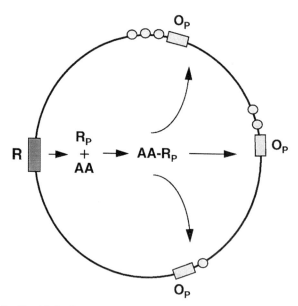

Figure 14–2. The Multiple-Operator Model (Regulon Model). A repressor molecule, R_p, whose synthesis depends on the gene R, combines with the amino acid AA whose synthesis is to be controlled. The repressor–amino acid complex, AA-R_p, binds to the operator DNA sequences, O_p, to prevent transcription of the genes within the three operons encoding for the enzymes of AA biosynthesis.

sor. In subsequent biochemical studies in the 1970s this was demonstrated to be the case. The regulon, in contrast to the operon, is a physiological unit, but not a genetic unit. Its component genes are not confined to a particular segment of DNA.

A refinement had to be introduced in the Operon Model when it was found that the site for binding of the repressor at O was not the same as the site at which the formation of messenger RNA by RNA polymerase was initiated. The latter site was called the promoter (P). Mutations in the promoter were found that prevented, as expected, the formation of beta-galactosidase and permease.

As mentioned above, the Operon Model is based exclusively on the lactose system and almost completely on genetic evidence. It is therefore not surprising that over the years, as more metabolic systems were studied, deviations from the Operon Model were found. These are discussed in Chapter 15. Most of the deviations occurred in the regulation of gene action. Striking differences were found in the way different pathways are regulated. Monod was a strong believer in a unitary hypothesis of regulation. As we have seen in the case of arginine and lactose, this belief was justified. However, later, as cases were found in which the mechanism of regulation was clearly different, Monod was always reluctant to accept such differences. He relied heavily on his intuition and convictions. As his colleague Irving Zabin put it, Monod, when learning of an experimental result that did not fit an idea of his would say, "I don't believe it for a minute."

In spite of the deviations found there are some features of the Operon Model that have remained constant, such as the promoter, the operator, and distinction between structural genes and regulatory genes. Thus, even with the existence of deviations, the Operon Model has had a great impact in directing the future of molecular genetics. It can be thought of as a framework for the construction of different kinds of buildings. Such buildings, having a common basic plan, may vary according to the final purpose for which they are constructed.

One topic that was not discussed at the 1961 Cold Spring Harbor Symposium was the genetic code. The reason for this omission is that the key experiment of Nirenberg and Matthei was carried out only a few weeks before the start of the Symposium. In fact, Nirenberg had applied to attend the Symposium, but was turned down. He had not published anything and he was unknown. The omission was rectified in the 1963 Cold Spring Harbor Symposium on "Synthesis and Structure of Macromolecules." At that time there were six talks on the genetic code, including one by Nirenberg.

. . .

We are now coming to the end of the period in the history of genetics that is the central part of this book. Its theme is the emergence of gene action in terms of defined chemical entities. In 1865, Mendel had a simple clear picture of gene action. He postulated the existence of separate elements, with each element determining a specific trait. These elements were transmitted independently from one generation to the next. By 1940, the picture was somewhat refined, with the elements now called genes, and the product of a gene being an enzyme responsible for the trait. The genes were still "black boxes." In the following 25 years, in a remarkable series of investigations, genes and their actions were analyzed chemically. The picture of gene action it gave us is precise, but it is also quite complicated. The gene has become part of a DNA molecule carrying the information for a protein molecule in the sequence of its base pairs. It transmits this information via messenger RNA to the protein-synthesizing machinery in the ribosomes. The most complicated part of gene action is its regulation. There is a start site for transcription of the gene by RNA polymerase, the promoter, and overlapping this site there is another site, the operator, where regulatory proteins, the products of regulatory genes, can bind and control the frequency at which transcription is initiated. "One gene–one enzyme" thus became a chemical reality.

The historian Horace Freeland Judson in his absorbing book entitled *The Eighth Day of Creation—Makers of the Revolution in Biology* refers to the period between 1940 and 1965 as a "Golden Age in Science." His book covers more or less the same period as I have done in my account but at much greater length and in much greater detail. Toward this end he interviewed 122 scientists (including myself) that he considered to be instrumental in the development of molecular genetics. He reported many of these interviews verbatim.

Judson asks the question, "What is a golden age like in science?" He considers one prerequisite for a golden age to be small groups of people coming from different disciplines, having intimate contact with each other. He states that "small size maximizes the collision frequency, the intensity of intellectual interactions; the variety of starting points maximizes the interplay, the scope, and angle of intersections of ideas." He goes further, however, by saying that, "a golden age in science is more than small size, modest needs, and big ideas. A true golden age is also an age of innocence. It thrives, for a while, in the competitive harsh ocean of the twentieth century, as an island of idealism, and of play, and of, at the same time, an austere devotion to intellectual enthusiasm and openness."

I like Judson's analysis of a golden age and I can testify to the points that he stresses. As an insider, I can confirm that it was an age of innocence. One aspect of science that was not apparent to me when I started in 1940 was the importance of science as an open communal effort. There were the great intellects who dominated the field by their style of leadership: Beadle, Delbrück, Crick, Monod, Lwoff; and there were the outstanding and original experimenters, Hotchkiss, Luria, Jacob, to name only a few. But I came to realize that their efforts would not have succeeded had it not been for the work done by the community of scientists as a whole and the frequent exchange of ideas.

I cannot express my feelings better than to quote the end of an autobiographical chapter written by the eminent biochemist Eugene Kennedy who worked in Lipmann's laboratory and later isolated the lactose permease protein. He relates a scientist's career to a poem by W.B. Yeats, entitled *Sailing to Byzantium,* and to me his interpretation of the poem incorporates the true spirit of science, as it was revealed during the period I have described.

The poem of Yeats is an ode that celebrates the works of art created by the soul of human beings. In interpreting the poem, Kennedy asks:

> What are these monuments of the soul's magnificence that we must study to transcend age and physical decay? Yeats meant the monuments of art, but surely there is another Byzantium to which we may sail and it contains the monuments of science. For those to whom fame is the spur, that last infirmity of noble minds, to labor on the monuments of art seems to hold a distinct advantage. Mozart, Beethoven, Yeats himself produced works that seem forever stamped with their personalities, like thumbprints on pottery. In contrast, scientists are interchangeable, with the rarest exceptions, perhaps none. The towering figure of Otto Warburg dominated biochemistry during the first half of this century. Today it is not easy to find a graduate student who can give a meaningful synopsis of his work.
>
> The anonymity that is the fate of nearly every scientist as the work of one generation blends almost without a trace into that of the next is a small price to pay for its unending progress, the great march of human reason. In his Nobel address, Fritz Lipmann said of scientists: "Their purpose often may be none but just to push back a little the limits of our comprehension. Their findings mostly have to be expressed in a scientific language that is understood only by a few. We feel, nevertheless, that the drive and urge to explore nature in all its facets is one of the most important functions of humanity." To feel that one has contributed to this splendid enterprise, on however small a scale, is reward enough for labor at the end of a day.

V

IN THE AFTERMATH
OF THE
OPERON MODEL,
1965–2000

I N 1965, the Operon Model had provided a concrete picture of gene action and its regulation as it occurred in the metabolism of *E. coli*. It showed us how the information encoded in the nucleotide sequence of DNA was transmitted via messenger RNA to produce enzyme molecules involved in metabolic reactions. Furthermore it showed us how this information transfer was controlled in response to external stimuli. The control was mediated by the products of other genes called regulatory genes. With this basic picture in mind, one could now turn to the action of genes in more complicated cellular processes, such as cell division and chromosome replication, and in other organisms, especially animals and plants. For the analysis of gene action one could use mutants as one had done with *E. coli*.

A priori, the fact that the Operon Model was based on work with *E. coli* suggested that it may apply only to bacteria. However, the founders of molecular genetics, who believed in the Unity of Biochemistry, were convinced that it would also apply to higher organisms (eukaryotes). Monod had asserted that what was true for *E. coli* would be true for the elephant. Crick had referred to *E. coli* as a eukaryote honoris causa.

Actually, the progress that was made between 1965 and the present time in the elucidation of gene action in eukaryotes is beyond the expectations of most people working in the field. This is mainly the result of the technological advances made in the handling of DNA. It became possible to carry out the same kind of analyses with eukaryotes as had previously been done with bacteria (prokaryotes). Although there are marked differences between prokaryotes and eukaryotes, nevertheless the previously established general view of gene action could be maintained and the Operon Model, as a framework, has survived as the paradigm of molecular genetics.

To relate the history described in the previous chapters to the present state of gene action, I give a brief account of the main advances since 1965. My intention is to connect the previously established roots with the spectacular developments of the past 35 years. It will become apparent at the end that the history of gene action is far from being finished and that much remains to be discovered, supporting the dictum that "science is an endless frontier."

15

The Floodgates Open

A DECISIVE factor in the rapid development of molecular genetics was the changes in the methodology from the cumbersome procedures of classical genetics involving the analysis of crosses, to chemical methods that make it possible to determine genetic characteristics directly and rapidly. These methods were introduced mainly by biochemists who, after 1965, entered the field in ever increasing numbers. Talks presented at meetings dealing with gene action were more and more in the province of chemistry.

The first major advance was the development of cloning methods in the early 1970s by S. Cohen and H. Boyer that eventually made it possible to study the expression of genes, either prokaryotic or eukaryotic, by transferring them to microorganisms. These methods were based on the use of certain enzymes, called restriction enzymes, that cut DNA at specific sites in the chromosome. One can insert such restriction enzyme fragments containing one or more genes into plasmids that serve as vectors for transferring these isolated genes into microorganisms, such as *E. coli*. The plasmids replicate in the microbial host. Most of the time the cloned genes in the plasmids are expressed in their new host and one can thus obtain not only large amounts of the cloned DNA, but also the proteins produced by the cloned genes. As an example, the human gene for insulin was cloned in this way and this led to the commercial production of human insulin.

The next major advance occurred in 1977 when two methods for sequencing DNA were published, one by A.M. Maxam and W. Gilbert, the other by F. Sanger and his associates. One could now determine without too much effort the coded information that is transmitted from one generation to the next. With the availability of this information and with the aid of the genetic code, the sequence of the encoded proteins can be deduced. This is much simpler than the protein sequencing method introduced previously by Sanger. The consequences resulting from the development of the two sequencing methods were enormous. To illustrate this, between 1965 and 1978 the sequences of DNA fragments containing a total of only 12,000 base pairs were published. In the next 4 years, about 1200 papers were published containing sequence data for over a million base pairs. Since then this number has approximately doubled every year. Central databases were established that stored the accumulated sequence information, which with the aid of computers could be analyzed for characteristic features, such as restriction enzyme sites, and which are accessible via computer networks to all investigators. The culmination of the sequencing technology was the development of automated methods, which made it possible to determine the DNA sequences of total genomes of many microorganisms, including *E. coli*, and yeast. The determination of the whole genome of higher organisms, such as *Drosophila*, mice, several plant species, and humans is well under way. The complete sequence of the *Drosophila* genome has been published in the 24 March 2000 issue of *Science*.

Several other methods were added that complemented or expanded the information obtained from sequencing data. One of these is the use of radioactively labeled DNA segments of known sequence as probes to detect the presence of genes in total DNA preparations. The method is based on the ability of the probe containing one strand of part of a known gene to hybridize with the complementary strand of this gene in the total DNA preparation. Such hybridized segments, usually deposited on a membrane, can be visualized by photographing the radioactive spots. In a similar fashion DNA probes can also be used for detecting specific messenger RNAs. In this way one can find out which genes in DNA are being transcribed. Recently this method has been automated and it is now possible to test simultaneously for the presence of thousands of messenger RNAs on a small piece of glass ("chip" method). One can thus determine which genes are turned on at different times in different parts of an organism.

A method that very much increases the sensitivity for detecting genes is the polymerase chain reaction (PCR), discovered by K. Mullis in 1985. It makes it possible to detect specific genes in single cells. The method is based on the amplification of DNA sequences where the sequence is known. By synthesizing short pieces of DNA that hybridize with the opposite ends or borders of a DNA segment, one can have them act as primers. The primers are extended toward the opposite border by an enzyme and many copies of the DNA segment are made. The process is called DNA amplification. The increase in the number of copies is exponential and in a short time millions of copies of a single gene can be generated. Understandably, this method has found wide applications, ranging from anthropology to medicine to criminal investigations.

Finally, simultaneously with the above-mentioned methods, several techniques were developed for altering base pairs of a DNA sequence in a defined way resulting in what is called site-specific mutagenesis. This has made it possible to determine the role of known base pairs in the functioning of a gene. The method has been particularly useful in conjunction with studies on the crystal structure of protein molecules in which specific amino acids have been altered. Using the genetic approach, one can test predictions made on the basis of the structural analysis. The approach is reminiscent of the previously described combination of genetic methods with cytological methods in the hybrid field of cytogenetics, except that now the level of analysis is at the molecular level rather than the level of structures visible under a microscope.

Regulation of Gene Action

In the history of biology there have always been two main approaches to research: a structural approach, carried out by anatomists and cytologists, and a functional approach, carried out by physiologists. The former gives qualitative pictures, the latter gives information about rates and dynamic interactions. Both approaches are essential. To illustrate this point for the history of gene action, we have seen that it was the structure of DNA that yielded a qualitative description, in the form of the genetic code, of the action of genes in determining the amino acid sequence of protein molecules. This was only part of the story. Following that, the studies on enzyme induction and enzyme repression provided a quantitative approach to gene action. It gave insight into the mechanism that controlled the rate of gene expression and it revealed the existence of regulatory genes. It was only after the combination of the two approaches that it was possible to construct a complete picture as formulated in the Operon Model. Studies since 1965 have concentrated on quantitative approaches to gene action, designed to investigate the regulatory mechanisms that make it possible for an organism to function as a harmonious whole under different conditions.

Prokaryotes

Since 1965 there has been an outburst of activities in the study of microbial metabolic pathways and their regulation. These studies have been expanded in breadth, with more and more metabolic systems being analyzed, and in depth, in penetrating the molecular details involved in regulatory mechanisms. The result has been the elucidation of diverse mechanisms of regulation in different pathways, with each pathway seemingly having found its own solution for satisfying its needs.

The earliest deviation from the Operon Model was the demonstration by Ellis Englesberg in the 1960s that the regulation of the formation of the enzymes involved in the utilization of the sugar arabinose were positively controlled. In this case, in contrast to the lactose repressor, the regulatory protein alone did not bind to the operator of the arabinose operon, yet the enzymes for arabinose breakdown were not produced. It was only after the binding of arabinose to the regulatory protein that the arabinose-protein complex bound to a site in the vicinity of the promoter and the enzymes were formed. It took several years for Englesberg to convince Monod of the validity of this positive control of enzyme formation. Similar positive control mechanisms were later demonstrated for the metabolic pathways of the sugars maltose and rhamnose.

In the 1970s a completely different mechanism of regulation was discovered, called attenuation, that depends not on the protein product of a regulatory gene being active at a promoter sequence but on the presence of codons for the amino acid whose production is being regulated near the beginning of the operon. This mechanism was first demonstrated in the biosynthesis of histidine where five histidine codons adjacent to each other occur at the beginning of the histidine operon DNA. In the presence of *high* concentrations of histidine the messenger RNA containing the five histidine codons is translated by ribosomes, which results in the formation of a "hairpin" structure called the attenuator in the messenger RNA. This, in turn, causes the termination of transcription of the operon and, subsequently prevents the formation of the histidine enzymes. In the presence of *low* concentrations of histidine translation is interrupted, the attenuator structure is not formed, and transcription of the operon proceeds normally. Such an attenuation mechanism has also been demonstrated in the biosynthesis of the amino acids phenylalanine, leucine, threonine, isoleucine, and tryptophan. In the last case, both a repressor protein mechanism and an attenuation mechanism are functional. These attenuation mechanisms have been studied mainly in *E. coli* and *Salmonella*, but they have also been found in other bacterial species.

Besides these regulatory mechanisms for specific metabolic pathways, higher-order regulatory mechanisms were found that affect many pathways. Regulatory proteins exerting this kind of control are called global regulators. One of the first global regulatory mechanisms, studied in the 1960s, was catabolite repression. A phenomenon underlying this regulation had first been noticed by Monod in the 1940s in his studies on the adaptive utilization of lactose, and was then called diauxie, as mentioned on page 113. Only later, when its general nature was realized, was it called catabolite repression. Monod showed that glucose was used in preference to lactose when both sugars were present. This seemed reasonable given that the utilization of glucose as an energy source involves a shorter, less energy-consuming chain of reactions than that of lactose and it is therefore advantageous for the bacteria to use glucose first. In the 1960s it was shown that the inhibition of lactose utilization by glucose was due to the lowering of the level of cyclic adenosine monophosphate (cAMP) in the cell. Derived from ATP, cAMP is a positive regulator of beta galactosidase that induces the formation of this enzyme. This is in addition to the lactose repressor, which inhibits enzyme formation. In the absence of cAMP, little enzyme is formed. In addition to cAMP a protein called CAP (catabolite activator protein) is required that binds to DNA near the promoter of the lactose operon and activates transcription, but only after cAMP is bound to it. This activating action of the CAP/cAMP complex was found not only in the utilization of lactose, but also in the utilization of other sugars such as galactose and arabinose. In more recent studies CAP/cAMP has been demonstrated to be involved as a regulator in about 70 different metabolic systems in *E. coli*. These included not only systems involved in the utilization of sugars and other carbon sources, but also in biosynthetic pathways and other cellular reactions. As is discussed later in this chapter it is also a global regulator in eukaryotes.

Several other global regulatory systems have been found in *E. coli* that are of similar complexity. A well-studied system of this kind involves the utilization of nitrogenous compounds, such as ammonia, glutamic acid, and glutamine as nitrogen sources for cellular growth. The result of having these global regulators complementing the action of repressors and inducers for individual pathways creates coordination among diverse cellular functions.

In addition to the successful analysis of many metabolic pathways, studies have also been carried out on the genes controlling timed cellular processes such as cell division and the replication of the chromosome and of plasmids. In these systems genes have been located that are required for these processes, but the mechanisms by which the action of these genes achieve their goals have not been elucidated so far. This remains a challenging subject for future studies.

Studies that probed in depth into the mechanism of regulation were centered on the structures of regulatory molecules, obtained by X-ray crystallography and NMR spectroscopy. Such studies are carried out by crystallographers, nowadays also called structural biologists. Of special interest is the mechanism by which the binding of an effector molecule, such as a sugar or an amino acid, to one site of a regulatory protein molecule can bring about a change in the binding to the DNA operator at another site of the protein molecule. This is what Monod called an allosteric transition.

Since 1965 a fair number of the regulatory proteins have been crystallized and their structures have been determined. In these structures the positions of all the atoms within the molecule are known. An outstanding example is the study of the Lac repressor, originally isolated by Gilbert and Müller-Hill. The crystal structure of the repressor has been determined recently by Mitchell Lewis, both by itself and when bound to either operator DNA or to the inducer isopropyl-thio-galactoside (IPTG). The repressor molecule consists of three regions: a core region, which is the binding site for the inducer; a headpiece, which is the binding site for DNA; and a flexible hinge, which connects the core to the headpiece. In the absence of inducer, the headpiece, which has two prongs, clasps the operator binding site like a pair of tweezers. When inducer binds to the core it changes the configuration of the whole molecule and a movement in the hinge brings about the opening of the prongs of the headpiece. The RNA polymerase enzyme, which transcribes the Lactose Operon, binds to DNA in the same region as the headpiece of the repressor and is held in place by the repressor. When the prongs open, RNA polymerase is released and can start the transcription of the lactose genes. This extraordinary analysis enables one to see the processes of repression and induction at the level of the atoms involved. This picture has been verified by complementary studies with 4042 mutants, isolated and mapped by Jeffrey Miller, that alter different base pairs of the repressor molecule and the operator site. In all these mutants, the effect of the mutation on the biological activity of the repressor is consistent with the expected change in the X-ray structure. In this case, the collaboration of Lewis, the structural biologist with Miller, the geneticist has led to a profound understanding of a regulatory process.

Eukaryotes

The eukaryotic genome is structurally and functionally much more complex than the prokaryotic genome. It is therefore not surprising that its regulation of gene action should also be more elaborate.

In regard to structure, the genome is housed in a structurally defined nucleus, surrounded by a membrane. The DNA in the nucleus exists as a complex with basic proteins, called histones. Because of its staining properties the complex is known as chromatin. It is organized into DNA-histone units, called nucleosomes. At a certain stage in the cell cycle, chromatin condenses to form the chromosomes. It is at this stage that mitosis occurs and the chromosomes divide.

At the molecular level, DNA segments coding for a protein are frequently interrupted by noncoding regions. Following transcription into messenger RNA, these noncoding regions are excised from the RNA before translation into a protein molecule occurs. The coding regions in DNA are called exons, the noncoding regions, introns.

In regard to function, in multicellular eukaryotic organisms, cells differentiate into many different types during development, whereas in prokaryotes, populations of cells belonging to the same species, with the exception of spore formation, remain fairly homogeneous. The information for carrying out differentiation is contained in the nucleotide sequence of the genome. Given that in most cases the complete genome is transmitted to all cells during development, differentiation must be due to activation and inactivation of different genes.

Initiation of transcription by RNA polymerase in eukaryotes occurs at promoters as it does in prokaryotes. However, the regulation of transcription is very different. Most of the DNA is present in the nucleosomes. Because of the coiling of DNA around histones in these structures, transcription of all genes is repressed except for those whose transcription is brought about by specific regulatory mechanisms. The presence of nucleosomes then establishes a zero baseline for transcription.

The first step in bringing about gene transcription is the removal of the repressive effect of nucleosomes. This is achieved by a group of enzymes that add acetate to the histones in the nucleosome. In addition to these acetylating enzymes, another group of proteins that remodel the chromatin complex is required for removal of repression.

Once promoters are freed of the repressive effect of nucleosomes they can interact with polymerase and initiate transcription. However, this process is controlled further by a large number (20–30) of proteins called transcription factors. Some of these bind to DNA near the initiation site and interact with RNA polymerase directly in initiating transcription. Others have specific DNA binding sites further upstream of the initiating site and function by increasing the efficiency of initiation. Some of these transcription factors are inducible by agents in the environment and are therefore produced only at specific times or in specific tissues. They are responsible for the establishment of changing transcription patterns that occur during cellular differentiation.

Besides the binding sites for transcription factors that are located in the vicinity of the promoter, there are other binding sites for transcription factors that are located at considerable distances from the promoter, on either side of the start site. These are called enhancers. Transcription factors that bind at enhancers interact with the proteins bound near the promoter and in this way affect transcription.

The inhibitory effect of chromatin on promoter function and, consequently gene expression is very stable and is transmitted from generation to generation. Since it does not involve changes in the DNA sequence, it is referred to as epigenetic control. It has also been called genetic imprinting. Epigenetic controls of varying degrees of permanence are common in eukaryotes and play major roles in the control of gene expression. A striking example is the dosage compensation to make up for the difference in the number of X-chromosomes in males and females. In *Drosophila* and in mammals there is one X-chromosome in the male and two X-chromosomes in females. In *Drosophila*, compensation is achieved by epigenetically stimulating transcription twofold in the male X-chromosome. In contrast, in mammals, X-linked gene expression is epigenetically equalized between the sexes by X-inactivation, the transcriptional silencing of one X-chromosome in female cells. This inactivation occurs early in embryonic development and persists throughout life.

Regulation and Development

Until the advent of regulatory genes in the mid-1950s, genetics and embryology, the study of development, proceeded along separate paths. Each field had its own methodology. Embryologists ignored genes. With the realization that there are genes that can turn on or turn off the activities of other genes, it became possible to visualize how such genes could bring about differentiation of cells during development without a change in their genetic constitution. This realization drew geneticists and embryologists together, as shown by a symposium held in 1958 with the title, "The Chemical Basis of Development." During this symposium several investigators, including myself, who were studying the control of enzyme synthesis, presented their work and tried to convince the embryologists who were present, how these controls could bring about cellular differentiation.

During the 1961 Cold Spring Harbor Symposium the same theme was voiced in very definite terms by Jacob and Monod. They raised the question whether cellular regulation and differentiation in higher organisms uses the same basic regulatory mechanisms as bacteria. The problem was that regulatory processes in bacteria are reversible, whereas processes involved in differentiation of higher organisms are largely irreversible. To overcome this dilemma, they constructed several models of interlocking regulatory circuits in which the interactions among repressors or inducers could bring about irreversible changes. There was now at least the theoretical possibility that bacterial regulatory mechanisms could account for differentiation.

In genetic studies carried out since 1965, the general notion that differentiation operates at the level of DNA by turning on or turning off transcription of genes has been confirmed, but the level of complexity was greater than anything envisaged by Jacob and Monod. Several model organisms have been used: the mouse, a worm called *Caenorhabditis elegans*, the zebrafish, and especially, the fruit fly *Drosophila*. The most detailed picture has been obtained from studies on mutants of *Drosophila* carried out by E.B. Lewis, C. Nüsslein-Vollhard, and E. Wieschaus. The three were awarded a Nobel Prize in 1995. As shown in the following paragraphs, their work illustrates the great complexity of interlocking genetic controls underlying development from egg to adult.

The development of *Drosophila* has been analyzed by isolating mutants that affect different stages of development and studying at the molecular level the functions that have been affected by the mutations. Three sets of genes were identified: maternal genes that control properties of the egg important in early development; segmentation genes that determine the number and location of segments in the fly's body (there are three thoracic segments and eight abdominal segments), and homeotic genes that control the structural characteristics of each segment.

Homeotic genes are arranged in the same order in the chromosome as the order of segments they control along the anterior–posterior axis of the fly's body. There is a hierarchy in the activity of these genes in that the deletion of a gene will result in the taking over of the activity of the deleted gene by the gene located anterior to it. For example, there is a homeotic gene that determines structures called halteres that are little knobs behind the wings. Anterior to it, there is a homeotic gene that determines the wings. Mutations that eliminate the activity of the gene for halteres have been shown to result in the production of flies with an extra pair of wings, in place of the halteres.

Many of the genes controlling development were found to determine the production of transcription factors that act on the expression of other genes. Overall, there is a cascade of gene actions, with genes in each group successively defining the properties of increasingly more restricted parts of the embryo. The maternal genes define broad regions in the egg; differences in the distribution of maternal gene products within the fertilized egg control the expression of segmentation genes. Once the segments are laid down, the homeotic genes are turned on to determine the details of each segment. The whole system is an intricate series of cascades with regulatory devices inserted at each level, so that the production of normal adults is insured.

An amusing feature is the naming of the *Drosophila* genes affecting development. The names are usually descriptive of the appearance of mutants. Since many of these mutants were isolated in Nüsslein-Vollhard's laboratory, the names are sometimes in German. Examples of names for maternal genes are: torpedo, gurken (cucumber), cactus, pipe, windbeutel (cream puff), nudel (noodle); for segmentation genes: hunchback, knirps (dwarf), even skipped, sloppy paired, gooseberry, hedgehog, disheveled.

Although the mechanics of development in terms of cellular events differ in detail in other species that have been studied, such as the mouse, the principles established with *Drosophila* seem to hold in the other cases: that a regulatory cascade determines the appropriate pattern of gene expression in cells of the embryo and ultimately of the adult. This notion is strengthened by the finding that homeotic genes are very similar in different species, including mice, worms and humans, and play similar roles in laying down structures of the body during the development of these organisms.

Application to Human Disease

As molecular genetics expanded after 1965 it began to make inroads into fields of practical importance, such as medicine, agriculture, and the pharmaceutical industry. Genetic engineering became a part of industrial developments. In all of these applications of genetics an understanding of gene action is important, but in none as much as in medicine. After a genetic change has been identified as the cause of a disease, it is imperative to know what this gene does before one can think of ways to cure the disease.

As an added benefit, the study of human diseases may lead, in reverse, to a better understanding of gene action. This was illustrated early by Garrod's work on diseases causing defects in amino acid metabolism that suggested the one gene–one enzyme hypothesis, and Pauling's work on sickle-cell hemoglobin that demonstrated a structural change in a protein molecule as a result of a mutation. Currently, about 10,000 genetic diseases have been registered and with the medical importance of these diseases stimulating research into their causes, new facts about gene action are bound to be discovered.

Mutations causing diseases have been shown to occur not only in structural genes but also in regulatory genes and in promoter sites where regulatory proteins act. In hemoglobin abnormalities known as thalassemias the mutations are located in the promoter of the hemoglobin gene. In a rare disease, called *xeroderma pigmentosum*, that renders patients very sensitive to ultraviolet light, the mutation is located in a transcription factor controlling a gene that normally produces an enzyme for the repair of DNA that has been damaged by ultraviolet light. Altogether, about 40 genetic diseases have been identified in which the mutation causes a defect in the production of a transcription factor.

A very active field of recent research has been the application of genetics to the study of infectious diseases. Such studies have concentrated on the genetic mechanisms of bacteria that are responsible for their pathogenicity, that is, their ability to produce disease. Pathogenic bacteria carry specialized genes that enable them to grow in a human (or animal) host and the products of these genes frequently cause damage to the host. For example, *E. coli* is a normal inhabitant of the human intestine, but there are strains of *E. coli* that have acquired genes that render them pathogenic. Frequently these genes are located in a plasmid that can be transmitted by mating (see page 89) or by transduction (see page 51) from one bacterium to another. For example, there is a gene that is responsible for the production of a toxin that causes diarrhea. Other genes are responsible for the ability of the bacteria to destroy intestinal cells, also causing diarrhea. Yet other genes cause changes in the surface structure of the bacteria that interfere with the natural defense mechanisms, such as antibodies, of the host. The genes responsible for pathogenesis are usually turned on by factors or conditions present in the host. For example, the gene for toxin production in *E. coli* is turned on the elevated temperature (37°C) inside the intestine.

The most spectacular impact of genetics on medicine has been the recognition that cancer is essentially a genetic disease. Although the frequency of inherited cancers is quite low—about 5% of all cancers—most cancers are the result of mutations or epigenetic changes that occur somewhere in the body of an organism and that are not transmitted to the offspring. For each type of cancer a series of such changes has to occur before the cancer begins to grow. For this reason, mutations that increase mutation frequency can be indirectly carcinogenic, as has been demonstrated for such mutations being responsible for colon cancer.

Cancer is initiated when an ordinarily quiescent cell starts to grow in an uncontrolled fashion. It is therefore not surprising that mutations responsible for cancer frequently occur in genes that function in the control of growth. Some of these genes code for transcription factors that regulate the activity of genes active in growth control. Transcription factors are, in turn, frequently controlled by external substances via signal transduction pathways that encompass several reactions. Mutations affecting these reactions may also cause cancer by affecting the action of a transcription factor. Since the branch of medicine dealing with cancer is called oncology, genes that are involved in production of cancer are call oncogenes. It is obvious that an understanding of the action of oncogenes is important for designing a rational treatment of cancer.

The Brain

The developments in embryology and medicine we have been considering were in fields that after 1965 were singled out as targets for future studies. The goals that were set at that time have been pursued vigorously and by now have led to a more profound understanding of the role of genes in these fields. Somewhat later, during the 1970s another area of biology, neurobiology, began to attract the attention of some molecular geneticists. It was the function of the brain that attracted their interest. At the beginning, genetic aspects were of only peripheral concern, but in more recent years they have assumed a more central position.

Francis Crick was one of the first molecular geneticists to switch from the gene to the brain. He tried to find an explanation for the nature of consciousness on the basis of what is known about the anatomy and physiology of the brain. In 1994 he described his ideas in the book *The Astonishing Hypothesis. The Scientific Search for the Soul*. He did not arrive at a final answer for the nature of consciousness, but, as in his work on the nature of the gene, he took the mysteries out of the problem. As he stated in the Preface of his book: "I am not at the moment enthusiastic about the views of functionalists, behaviorists, and some physicists, mathematicians and philosophers . . . Now is the time to think scientifically about consciousness (and its relationship, if any, to the hypothetical immortal soul) and, most importantly of all, the time to start the *experimental* study of consciousness in a serious and deliberate way."

The person who introduced experimental genetics into the study of the brain (and the mind) is Seymour Benzer (Fig. 15–1). In the 1960s he switched from bacteriophages to *Drosophila* and set up a "flyroom" at Cal Tech. His aim was to isolate mutants in which behavior was altered. He assumed that a hereditary change in behavior must have changed a gene that codes for a molecular com-

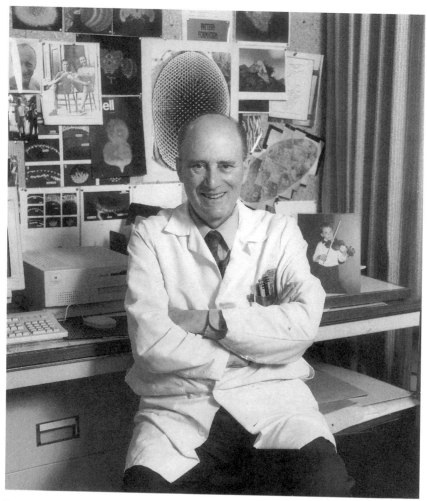

FIGURE 15–1. Seymour Benzer in his office at Caltech. [Courtesy of Seymour Benzer.]

ponent involved in producing that behavior. He designed several ingenious methods for the selection of such mutants and soon began to isolate them. The mutants that he and his associates found were affected in various aspects of behavior. As in the case of developmental mutants, they received unusual names. For example, they isolated mutants with defects in learning and memory. They were named dunce, rutabaga, amnesiac, and linotte. The mutations were mapped. Later, biochemical studies showed that they were defective at different steps of the signal transduction pathway that connects cAMP with a transcription factor called CREB (cyclic AMP response element binding protein). Since the mutants were defective in the conversion of short-term memory to long-term memory, it was concluded that the promoter controlled by CREB is linked to genes that function in this process.

Other mutants showed differences in sexual behavior. Male mutants unable to mate successfully were named celibate and coitus interruptus. A homosexual male mutant was named fruitless. A mutant with a defective sense of time was named timeless and a mutant that could not tell the temperature was named bizarre.

Similar studies on behavioral mutants have been carried out with mice. In these studies, cAMP also was found to be implicated in some of the mutations.

The work on behavioral mutants is at the frontier of studies on gene action. How genes control the functioning of the brain is a largely unexplored field. It is an exciting prospect for the future that by pursuing these studies we may eventually be able to understand how our brains function and what limits are set by our genes to our mental capabilities.

The Current Status of Gene Action

Having reached the end of my account of the history of gene action I look back on the picture that has emerged after a hundred years of investigations.

The genes themselves are stretches of DNA that contain the information encoded in their sequences for carrying out all the activities of living cells. This information is transmitted from generation to generation. It determines the capabilities and limitations of living organisms.

The primary action of genes is to produce messenger RNA molecules which, in turn, give rise to protein molecules or, in some cases, RNA molecules, such as transfer RNAs or ribosomal RNAs. Besides specific coding regions, there are other regions preceding and following the coding region (leaders and trailers) and, in the case of eukaryotes, intervening sequences (introns) between individual coding segments (exons). At the start of the leading region there is a promoter sequence that serves as the binding site for RNA polymerase to initiate transcription.

There are two kinds of genes, structural genes and regulator genes. The former are concerned with determining the structural and enzymatic components of cells. The latter regulate the activities of genes, including their own transcription. Three kinds of regulatory genes can be distinguished: (*1*) those involved in the regulation of specific metabolic pathways; (2) global regulatory genes that bring about coordination among different pathways; and (3) genes that act on the conformation and structure of DNA, resulting in permanent effects on the expression of genes contained in DNA. This leads to what is called epigenetic inheritance or gene imprinting.

Regulation of gene action is frequently brought about by environmental influences. Such environmental effects are transmitted via signal pathways to proteins called transcription factors that act on promoters to regulate the initiation of gene transcription. In some cases they inhibit transcription; in others, they stimulate it.

As the analysis of gene action and its regulation has progressed, the picture has become more and more complicated, especially during the past 30 years. Today we are confronted with an intricate array of biochemical processes that occur between the primary gene action and the final phenotype. Disentangling these complicated interactions can be a frustrating task, but it is necessary to carry it out if we want to achieve control over these processes. Nowadays a great deal of publicity is given to the importance of sequencing genomes, especially the human genome. It should be clear from what has been said that knowledge of gene sequences is very valuable, because it contains all the information for assembling an organism. However, this information is written in the language of the genetic code, and we have a long way to go before we shall be able to follow the instructions contained in the coded messages to their final destination in the construction of an organism. This enormous task is the subject of future research.

APPENDIX

Further Readings and Comments

My aim is to provide the reader with references that will enable him or her to follow-up on topics discussed in the text. Most of the references are to key books and articles in journals. The latter are listed by title and author, followed by the name of the journal, volume number, first and last page numbers, and the year of publication (in parentheses). The cited books and articles frequently provide listings of significant earlier publications.

Some of the articles cited in the following sections have been collected into a bound volume. Cited papers present in these volumes are marked by the letter preceding the title of the books listed below.

A. *Classic Papers in Genetics.* Edited by James A. Peters. Prentice-Hall, Englewood Cliffs, NJ (1959).
B. *Papers of Bacterial Genetics.* Selected by Edward A. Adelberg. Little, Brown and Company, Boston, MA (1960).
C. *Papers on Bacterial Viruses.* Selected by Gunther S. Stent. Little, Brown and Company, Boston, MA (1960).
D. *The Molecular Basis of Life.* Readings from Scientific American, W.H. Freeman and Company, San Francisco, CA (1968).

Preface

The two books mentioned in the Preface give authoritative accounts of the Classical Period between 1860 and 1940. The references are: *A Short History of Genetics*, by L.C. Dunn. New York: McGraw-Hill (1965) and *A History of Genetics*, by A.H. Sturtevant. New York: Harper and Row (1965). The developments during this period are also covered in the textbook: *An Introduction to Genetics*, by A.H. Sturtevant and G.W. Beadle. Philadelphia; W.B. Saunders Company (1940).

Chapter 1

Detailed descriptions of Mendel are provided by the biographies of Hugo Iltis (*The Life of Mendel*. Translated by Eden and Cedar Paul. New York: Hafner Publishing Co., 1966) and Vitezslav Orel (*Gregor Mendel: The First Geneticist*. Translated by Stephen Finn. Oxford University Press, 1996). Iltis grew up in Brno and became a teacher at the local high school. He was very familiar with Mendel's life and career and relating Mendel's history became his major occupation. Being Jewish, he was forced to leave Brno during the Nazi Period and he settled in Fredericksburg, Virginia and became the curator of the Mendel Museum. Orel was until a few years ago the Head of the Mendelianum (Mendel museum) in Brno and has been very active in studying and publicizing Mendel's heritage. Another more popular account was published recently, *Gregor Mendel and the Roots of Genetics*, by Edward Edelson (New York: Oxford University Press, 1999). It gives an overview not only of Mendel's career, but also of the subsequent suppression of Mendelian Genetics by Russian communism and of the emergence of molecular genetics.

A good introduction to Mendel's work and legacy is provided by a website, called **MendelWeb,** http://www.netspace.org/MendelWeb/. It contains Mendel's original papers (in German) and English translations and much biographical material. It also contains a delightful article, "In the Footsteps of Mendel," by Margaret Peaslee, describing her recent visit to the Mendelianum and to Mendel's birthplace. But foremost, it contains two articles by Jan Sapp ("The Nine Lives of Gregor Mendel") and Robert C. Olby ("Mendel, Mendelism and Genetics") that deal with the (sometimes opposing) interpretations of the significance of Mendel's work. These publications seem to raise questions about the greatness of Mendel's contribution as the founding father of genetics. Fortunately, two recent articles (not in **MendelWeb**) seem to affirm Mendel's original stature. They are: "What Did Gregor Mendel Think He Discovered" by Daniel Hartl and Vitezslav Orel, (*Genetics, 131:* 245–253, June 1992) and "Development: Mendel's Legacy to Genetics," by Iris Sandler (*Genetics, 154:* 7–11, January 2000).

The aspect of Mendel's work that is of special relevance to gene action was his recognition of unitary elements (now called genes) that determine specific characteristics. This contribution of Mendel was ignored for a long time. Around 1950 it was finally recognized. In a memorial volume for the first 50 years of genetics, *Genetics in the 20th Century*, edited by L.C. Dunn (New York: The Macmillan Company, 1951), the cytogeneticist C.D. Darlington in a lecture entitled "Mendel and the Determinants" stated that "it has taken 50 years to rediscover the determinants which he called elements and which we call genes." At another point he stated that "the name of genetics which Bateson gave to this science announced to the world their (the early Mendelians) belief in the tremendous implications of what seemed to the impartial by-stander to be mere statistical trivialities. That belief we now know has been justified by 50 years of inquiry—but not in the way they expected. For in this time the elements have superseded the ratios." To paraphrase Darlington, by 1950 Mendel was not only the father of the Rules of Inheritance, but also the Father of Gene Action.

Chapter 2

The papers describing the three independent rediscoveries of Mendel's work by Hugo De Vries, Carl Correns, and Erich Tschermak were published in English translation in a supplement to the journal *Genetics* (Volume 35, September 1950). This supplement also contains Mendel's letters to Carl Nägeli (in translation), written between 1866 and 1873. A similar collection was published in book form by Curt Stern and Eva R. Sherwood, entitled *The Origin of Genetics. A Mendel Source Book* (San Francisco: W.H. Freeman and Company, 1966). This book is recommended because it contains a critical introduction and new and more discerning translations of the original papers.

An excellent account of the chromosomal basis of inheritance is provided in the book: *The Chromosome Theory of Inheritance: Classic Papers in Development and Heredity.* Edited by Bruce R. Voeller, New York: Appleton-Century-Crofts (1968). Further accounts are given in the previously mentioned histories by Dunn and Sturtevant, in *The Cell in Development and Heredity* by Edmund B. Wilson, New York: The Macmillan Company, Third Edition (1925), and in *Heredity and Development*, by John A. Moore, New York: Oxford University Press (1963). The quoted statement by de Vries is cited in Dunn's book, *A Short History of Genetics*, on page 43. In the previously mentioned book, *Genetics in the 20th Century*, there are relevant chapters by H.J. Muller: "The Development of the Gene Theory" and by A.H. Sturtevant: "The Relations of Genes and Chromosomes." Outstanding experimental papers by Sturtevant on the mapping of genes and by Muller on the induction of mutations are in volume (A) of the Collected Papers. This volume contains also the classical paper by Walter S. Sutton: "The Chromosomes in Heredity," published in the *Biological Bulletin, 4:* 231–251 (1903).

A description of the Morgan School and its successors is presented in *Lords of the Fly,* by Robert E. Kohler, Chicago: The University of Chicago Press (1994). It tells all one wants to know about *Drosophila* and its protagonists.

Books that deal with biochemical studies of DNA during the Classical Period are: *Molecules and Life,* by Joseph S. Fruton, New York: Wiley Interscience (1972); *A Century of DNA,* by F.H. Portugal and J.S. Cohen, MIT Press (1977); and *The Path to the Double Helix,* by Robert Olby, University of Washington Press (1974).

A comprehensive overview of both genetic and biochemical studies during the Classical Period is presented in an article by Bentley Glass: "A Century of Biochemical Genetics," in *The Proceedings of the American Philosophical Society, 109:* 227–236 (1965).

Chapters 3 and 4

The references for these two chapters have been combined because they deal with the same subject, the action of genes in the control of enzyme formation.

The 1903 contribution of Cuenot to the one gene—one enzyme concept, published in a paper entitled: "Hypothèse sur l'Hérédité des Couleurs dans les Croisements des Souris Noires, Grises et Blanches," *Com. Rend. Soc. Biol., 55:* 301–302 (1903), has been critically evaluated by R.P. Wagner: On the Origins of the Gene–Enzyme Hypothesis, *Journal of Heredity, 80:* 503–504 (1989). A good account of Garrod's work is given in a book by H. Harris, entitled *Garrod's Inborn Errors of Metabolism.* London: Oxford University Press (1963). This book contains the six Croonian Lectures delivered in 1908, a paper on alkaptonuria, entitled: "The Incidence of Alkaptonuria: A Study in Chemical Individuality," by Archibald E. Garrod, *Lancet, 2:* 1616 (1902), and a complete bibliography of Garrod's writings.

The notion that genes control the production of enzymes is also expounded in Bateson's book, *Mendel's Principles of Heredity,* New York; G.P. Putnam's Sons (1909), in Wright's paper, "Color Inheritance in Mammals," *Journal of Heredity, 8:* 224–235 (1917) and in Goldschmidt's paper, "Genetic Factors and Enzyme Reaction," *Science, 43:* 98–100 (1916). Haldane's ideas on this subject are discussed in his two books, *New Paths in Genetics,* New York: Harper and Bros. (1942) and *The Biochemistry of Genetics,* New York, Macmillin (1954). His work and his ideas on the same subject are also reviewed in a chapter by Ernst Caspari in a memorial volume, entitled *Haldane and Modern Biology,* Baltimore: The Johns Hopkins Press (1968).

The studies of Beadle and Ephrussi on *Drosophila* eye pigments are described in the previously mentioned book, *Lords of the Fly,* by Robert E. Kohler. They are also reviewed in an article by Norman Horowitz: "The Origins of Molecular Genetics: One Gene, One Enzyme." *Bio Essays, 3:* 37–39 (1981). The methodology is described in a paper, entitled: "A Technique of Transplantation of *Drosophila,*" by Boris Ephrussi and G.W. Beadle. *American Naturalist, 70:* 217–225 (1936).

The work of the *Neurospora* group is described in a classic review article by Beadle, entitled: "The Genes of Men and Molds," in *Scientific American,* September 1948, reprinted in (D). It is also described in the aforementioned article by Norman Horowitz, as well as in another article by him, entitled: "Fifty

Years Ago: The *Neurospora* Revolution." *Genetics, 127:* 631–635 (1991); Beadle has described their work in a *Harvey Lecture:* "The Genetic Control of Biochemical Reactions," *Harvey Lectures Series, 40:* 179–194 (1944–45). The 1941 paper by Beadle and Tatum, "Genetic Control of Biochemical Reactions in *Neurospora*," appeared in *The Proceedings of the National Academy of Sciences, 27:* 499–506 (1941) reprinted in (A).

Neurospora is described in a review article, entitled: "*Neurospora:* The Organism Behind the Molecular Revolution," by David D. Perkins, *Genetics, 130:* 687–701 (1992).

Chapter 5

Much of the material of this chapter and of some of the subsequent chapters (6, 7, 12, 13, 14) is covered in the book: *The Emergence of Bacterial Genetics*, by Thomas D. Brock, Cold Spring Harbor Laboratory Press (1990). An excellent collection of articles by the founders of molecular genetics and dealing for the most part with microbes can be found in *Phage and the Origins of Molecular Biology*, edited by John Cairns, Gunther S. Stent, and James D. Watson, Cold Spring Harbor Laboratory of Quantitative Biology (1966). These essays are dedicated to Max Delbrück on the occasion of his 60th birthday.

The contributions of Beijerinck are reviewed in Brock's book. A more comprehensive account is given in: *Martinus Willem Beijerinck, His Life and His Work*, by G. Van Iterson Jr. , L.E. Den Dooren De Jong, and A.J. Kluyver, The Hague: Martinus Nijhoff (1940). This is in Volume VI of *Beijerinck's Collected Writings*.

A personal account of Luria's work is presented in his autobiography, *A Slot Machine, A Broken Test Tube*, New York; Harper and Row (1984). The classical paper describing the fluctuation test is entitled: "Mutations of Bacteria from Virus Sensitivity to Virus Resistance," by S.E. Luria and M. Delbrück, *Genetics, 28:* 491–511 (1943).

Lederberg has described his discovery of mating in *E. coli* in an article, entitled: "Genetic Recombination in Bacteria: A Discovery Account." *Annual Reviews of Genetics, 21:* 23–46 (1987). The first announcement of sexual recombination was in a note: "Gene Recombination in *Escherichia coli*," by Joshua Lederberg and Edward l. Tatum, *Nature, 158:* 558 (1946), reprinted in (A). The discovery of transduction was reported in the paper: "Genetic Exchange in *Salmonella*," by Norton D. Zinder and Joshua Lederberg, *Journal of Bacteriology, 64:* 679–699 (1952). The method of testing all colonies on an agar plate simultaneously for different characteristics was reported in the paper: "Replica Plating and Indirect Selection of Bacterial Mutants," by Joshua Lederberg and Esther M. Lederberg, *Journal of Bacteriology, 63:* 399–406 (1952), reprinted in (B).

Chapter 6

The penicillin enrichment method for the isolation of auxotrophic mutants was first described in two papers, "Isolation of Biochemically Deficient Mutants of Bacteria by Penicillin," by B.D. Davis. *Journal of the American Chemical Society.* 70: 4267 (1948), and "Concentration of Biochemical Mutants of Bacteria with Penicillin," by J. Lederberg and N.D. Zinder. *Journal of the American Chemical Society, 70:* 4267–4268 (1948). Further articles are: "Isolation and Characterization of Biochemical Mutants of Bacteria," by J. Lederberg. *Methods in Medical Research, 3:* 5–22 (1950), and "Studies on Nutritionally Deficient Bacterial Mutants Isolated by Means of Penicillin," by B.D. Davis, *Experientia, 6:* 41–50 (1950).

Much of the work of Davis' laboratory is summarized in "Biochemical Explorations with Bacterial Mutants," by B.D. Davis. *Harvey Lectures, 50:* 230–244 (1954–55). Mutationally altered enzymes are described in "Production of an Altered Pantothenate-Synthesizing Enzyme by a Temperature-Sensitive Mutant of *Escherichia coli*," by Werner K. Maas and Bernard D. Davis. *Proceedings of the National Academy of Sciences, 38:* 785–797 (1952), and, in the same issue, pages 775–785, "Analysis of the Biochemical Mechanism of Drug Resistance in Certain Bacterial Mutants," by Bernard D. Davis and Werner K. Maas.

The studies of Horowitz and Leupold are reported in the article: "Some Recent Studies Bearing on the One Gene–One Enzyme Hypothesis," by N.H. Horowitz and Urs Leupold. *Cold Spring Harbor Symposium on Quantitative Biology, 16:* 65–72 (1951), reprinted in (A).

The work on sickle cell hemoglobin was reported in a paper, entitled: "Sickle Cell Anemia: A Molecular Disease," by L. Pauling, H. Itano, S.J. Singer, and I.C. Wells. *Science, 110:* 543–548 (1949). The identification of the amino acid change in sickle-cell hemoglobin was described in a paper, entitled: "Gene Mutations in Human Hemoglobin: The Chemical Difference Between Normal and Sickle Cell Hemoglobin," by V.M. Ingram. *Nature, 180:* 326–328 (1957); reprinted in *The Journal of NIH Research, 7:* 53–57 (1995).

The paper of Edgar, describing the use of temperature-sensitive mutants is entitled: "Temperature-Sensitive Mutants of Bacteriophage T4D: Their Isolation and Genetic Characterization," by R.S. Edgar and I. Lielausis. *Genetics, 49:* 649–662 (1964).

Chapter 7

The story of the discovery of DNA is told by one of the codiscoverers in *The Transforming Principle,* by Maclyn McCarty. New York: W.W. Norton and Company (1985). The original paper is entitled: "Studies on the Chemical Nature of the Substance Inducing Transformation of Pneumococcal Types," by Oswald T. Avery, Colin M. MacLeod, and Maclyn McCarty, *Journal of Experimental Medicine, 79:* 137–158 (1944) (reprinted in A). McCarty published an article: "Reminiscences of the Early Days of Transformation," in *Annual Review of Genetics, 14:* 1–15 (1980).

Hotchkiss reviewed his work in an article, entitled: "The Identification of Nucleic Acids as Genetic Determinants," in the *Origins of Modern Biochemistry,* edited by P.R. Srinivasan, J.S. Fruton and J.T. Edsall. *Annals of the New York Academy of Sciences, 325:* 321–342 (1979).

Crucial evidence for DNA being the genetic material was provided in the paper: "Independent Functions of Viral Protein and Nucleic Acid in Growth of Bacteriophage," by A.D. Hershey and M. Chase. *Journal of General Physiology, 36:* 39–56 (1952), reprinted in (C).

The exciting story of solving the structure of DNA is described in vivid detail in: *The Double Helix,* by James D. Watson. New York: W.W. Norton and Company (1985).

The original paper: "Molecular Structure of Nucleic Acids," by J.D. Watson and F.H.C. Crick. *Nature, 171:* 737–738 (1953), is reprinted in (A). A report on the semiconservative replication of DNA appeared in the article: "The Replication of DNA," by M. Meselson, and F.W. Stahl, in *Cold Spring Harbor Symposia on Quantitative Biology, 23:* 9–12 (1958). Their original paper is in the *Proceedings of the National Academy of Sciences, 44:* 671–682 (1958).

Chapter 8

The studies on the theoretical basis of the genetic code are described in Crick's autobiography: *What Mad Pursuit,* by Francis Crick. New York: Basic Books, Inc. (1988). The early studies by Brachet and by Caspersson on the role of RNA in protein synthesis are well presented and documented in the book *The Biosynthesis of Proteins,* by H. Chantrenne, Oxford: Pergamon Press (1961). Brachet's contribution is remembered in an article entitled: "Molecular Genetics Under an Ambryologist's Microscope: Jean Brachet, 1909–1988," by René Thomas. *Genetics, 131:* 515–518 (1992). Gamow's scheme for a genetic code is described in a paper, entitled: "Possible Relation Between Deoxyribonucleic Acid and Protein Structure," in *Nature, 173:* 318 (1954). Brenner's paper disproving an overlapping code, is entitled: "On the Impossibility of all Overlapping Triplet Codes in Information Transfeer from Nucleic Acid to Protein," by S. Brenner, *Proceedings of the National Academy of Sciences, 43:* 687–694 (1957). Crick presented his adaptor hypothesis in a paper, entitled: "On Protein Syntehsis, by F.H.C. Crick." *Symposium of the Society of Experimental Biology, 12:* 138–163 (1958).

Sanger's discovery of a method for sequencing proteins is recounted in: "Protein Sequencing and the Making of Molecular Genetics," by Soraya De Chadarevian, *Trends in Biochemical Sciences* (*TIBS*), *24*: 203–206 (May 1999).

Chapter 9

The classical review article on the high-energy phosphate bond is entitled: "Metabolic Generation and Utilization of Phosphate Bond Energy," by Fritz Lipmann. *Advances of Enzymology, 1:* 99–162 (1941). The role of the high-energy phosphate bond in protein synthesis is discussed in an article, entitled: "On the Mechanism of Some ATP-Linked Reactions and Certain Aspects of Protein Synthesis," by F. Lipmann, pages 599–604, in *The Mechanisms of Enzyme Action.* Edited by W.D. McElroy and B. Glass Baltimore: The Johns Hopkins Press (1954). The quotation from Lipmann's article on page 128 is on page 241 in a book entitled: *Currents in Biochemical Research,* edited by D.E. Green. New York: Interscience Publishers (1956). The synthesis of pantothenic acid is described in "The Biosynthesis of Pantothenic Acid," by Werner K. Maas, *Fourth International Congress Of Biochemistry, Vol. II: Vitamin Metabolism,* pages 161–168, London: Pergamon Press (1959).

An overall view of the work in Zamecnik's laboratory is presented in the book: *Toward a History of Epistemic Things: Synthesizing Proteins in the Test Tube,* by Hans-Jörg Rheinberger. Stanford: Stanford University Press (1997). A review article by Zamecnik is entitled: "Historical Aspects of Protein Synthesis," in *Annals of the New York Academy of Sciences, 325:* 269–301 (1979). Transfer RNA is described in a paper, entitled: "A Soluble Ribonucleic Acid Intermediate in Protein Synthesis," by M.B. Hoagland, M.L Stephenson, J.F. Scott, L.I. Hecht, and P.C. Zamecnik. *Journal of Biological Chemistry, 231:* 241–257 (1958). Mahlon Hoagland has given an amusing account of his discovery, entitled: "Biochemistry or Molecular Biology? The Discovery of Soluble RNA," in *Trends in Biochemical Sciences* (*TIBS*), *21:* 77–80 (1996).

Chapter 10

The occasion leading to the recognition of messenger RNA is quoted from pages 119 and 120 of Crick's previously cited book, *What Mad Pursuit.* Two experimental papers demonstrating messenger RNA are entitled: "An Unstable Intermediate Carrying Information from Genes to Ribosomes for Protein Synthesis," by S. Brenner, F. Jacob, and M. Meselson. *Nature, 190:* 576–581 (1961), and Unstable Ribonucleic Acid Revealed by Pulse Labeling of *Escherichia coli,* by F. Gros, H. Hiatt, W. Gilbert, C.G. Kurland, R.W. Riseborough, and J.D. Watson. *Nature, 190:* 581–585 (1961). Brenner and Gros presented their work at the 1961 *Cold Spring Harbor Sympsoium of Quantitative Biology, Volume 26:* 101–110 (Brenner) and 111–132 (Gros) (1961).

The "Pajamo" experiment is described in a paper entitled: "The Genetic Control and Cytoplasmic Expression of 'Inducibility' in the Synthesis of β-Galactosidase by *E. coli*," by A.B. Pardee, F. Jacob and J. Monod. *Journal of Molecular Biology, 1:* 165–178 (1959). Decline of enzyme synthesis following the destruction of the gene during radioactive decay of its phosphorus atoms is described in a paper entitled: "On the Expression of a Structural Gene," by M. Riley, A.B. Pardee, F. Jacob, and J. Monod. *Journal of Molecular Biology, 2:* 216–225 (1960). A good background source for *E. coli* genetics is the excellent book: *The Genetics of Bacteria and Their Viruses*, by William Hayes. New York: John Wiley and Sons, Second Edition (1968).

Chapter 11

Several articles on the genetic code are reprinted in the volume, *The Molecular Basis of Life. Readings from the* Scientific American (D). They are: "The Genetic Code: II," by Marshall W. Nirenberg (March 1963). "The Genetic Code: III," by F.H.C. Crick (October 1966). An article on the related topic of colinearity between genes and proteins, entitled: "Gene Structure and Protein Structure," by Charles Yanofsky (May 1967). The book: *The Genetic Code*, by Carl R. Woese, New York: Harper and Row (1967), gives an authoritative summary of this topic.

The following papers in Volume 31 of the *Cold Spring Harbor Symposia on Quantitative Biology* (1966), entitled *The Genetic Code* are of special interest: "Polynucleotide Synthesis and the Genetic Code," by H.G. Korana, et al. (9 coworkers), pages 39–51. "Frameshift Mutations and the Genetic Code," by G. Streisinger, et al. (6 coworkers), pages 77–84. "Amino Acid Replacements and the Genetic Code," by Charles Yanofsky, Juetsu Ito, and Virginia Horn, pages 151–162. Genetic evidence for colinearity is presented in a paper, entitled: "Colinearity of the Gene with the Polypeptide Chain," by A.S. Sarabhai, A.O.W. Stretton and S. Brenner, *Nature, 201:* 13–17 (1964). The evidence for the anticodon site of transfer RNA determining the incorporation of an amino acid into the polypeptide chain is described in the paper "On the Role of Soluble Ribonucleic Acid in Coding for Amino Acids," by François Chapeville, Fritz Lipmann, Günter von Ehrenstein, Bernard Weisblum, William J. Ray, Jr., and Seymour Benzer. *Proceedings of the National Academy of Sciences, 48:* 1086–1092 (1962).

An account of Benzer's work is given in "Genetic Fine Structure," by Seymour Benzer, *Harvey Lectures, 56:* 1–21 (1961), and in "The Fine Structure of the Gene," by Seymour Benzer, *Scientific American* (January 1962) (reprinted in (D)).

Chapter 12

The studies on the regulation of arginine are reviewed in three papers in the previously cited *Cold Spring Harbor Symposium*, Volume 26 (1961). (*1*) "Aspects of Repression in the Regulation of Enzyme Synthesis: Pathway-wide Control and Enzyme-specific Response," by H.J. Vogel, pages 163–172. (*2*) "Genetics of Regulation of Enzyme Synthesis in the Arginine Biosynthetic Pathway of *Escherichia coli*," by L. Gorini, W. Gundersen, and M. Burger, pages 173–182. (*3*) "Studies on Repression of Arginine Biosynthesis in *Escherichia coli*," by W.K. Maas, pages 183–192. In the same volume, feedback control of enzyme activity is reviewed in "Feedback Control by Endproduct Inhibition," by H.E. Umbarger, pages 301–312.

The publication of the chemostat was in a paper, entitled: "Description of the Chemostat," by A. Novick and L. Szilard, *Nature, 112:* 715–716 (1950).

Clustering of genes of biosynthetic pathways was reviewed in "Complex Loci in Microorganisms," by M. Demerec and P.E. Hartman, *Annual Review of Microbiology, 13:* 377–406 (1959). Coordinate control of enzyme synthesis in a biosynthetic pathway was described in a paper, entitled: "Coordinate Repression of the Synthesis of Four Histidine Biosynthetic Enzymes by Histidine," by Bruce N. Ames and Barbara Garry. *Proceedings of the National Academy of Sciences, 45:* 1453–1461 (1959).

The allosteric mechanism underlying feedback control of enzyme activity is described in two papers: (*1*) "The Enzymology of Control by Feedback Inhibition," by John C. Gerhart and Arthur B. Pardee, *The Journal of Biological Chemistry, 237:* 891–896 (1962). (*2*) "Allosteric Proteins and Cellular Control Systems," by Jaques Monod, Jean-Pierre Changeux, and François Jacob. *Journal of Molecular Biology, 6:* 306–329 (1963).

An overview of the regulation of amino acid biosynthesis is provided in the book *Amino Acids: Biosynthesis and Genetic Regulation,* by Klaus M. Herrman and Ronald L. Somerville. Addison-Wesley Publishing Company, Advanced Book Program, Reading, Massachusetts (1983).

Chapter 13

Monod has described the history leading to the lactose operon in his Nobel lecture: "From Enzymatic Adaptation to Allosteric Transition," in *Science, 154:* 476–483 (1966). The "Pajamo" paper is listed in the references for Chapter 10.

An account leading to the conclusion that enzyme induction is the reversal of enzyme repression is given in "The Regulation of Arginine Biosynthesis: Its Contribution to Understanding the Control of Gene Expression," by Werner K. Maas. *Genetics, 128:* 489–494 (1991). The isolation and genetic properties of F⁻ prime factors, such as F-lac, are described in a short paper, entitled "Transfer of Genetic Characters by Incorporation in the Sex Factor of *Escherichia coli*," by François Jacob and Edward A. Adelberg, *Comptes Rendus des Séances de l'Académie des Sciences, 249:* 189–191 (1959). English translation in (B).

Chapter 14

The account of the lactose operon is in the previously cited *Cold Spring Harbor Symposium,* Volume 26 (1961) in the article: "On the Regulation of Gene Activity," by F. Jacob and J. Monod, pages 193–212. Expanded accounts are presented in the review article, "Genetic Regulatory Mechanisms in the Synthesis of Proteins," by François Jacob and Jaques Monod, *Journal of Molecular Biology, 3:* 318–356 (1961), and in Jacob's Nobel lecture: "Genetics of the Bacterial Cell," *Science, 152:* 1470–1478 (1966). Subsequent developments are described in the book *The Lactose Operon,* edited by Jonathan R. Beckwith and David Zipser. Cold Spring Harbor Laboratory Press (1970).

The regulon model was proposed in a paper, entitled: "Studies on the Mechanism of Repression of Arginine Biosynthesis in *Escherichia coli:* Dominance of Repressibility in Diploid," by W.K. Maas and A.J. Clark. *Journal of Molecular Biology, 8:* 365–370 (1964).

An excellent overall view over the emergence of molecular genetics is given by Horace Freehand Judson in *The Eighth Day of Creation—Makers of the Revolution in Biology,* Expanded edition, Cold Spring Harbor Press (1996).

Chapter 15

Some recent books and reviews are listed for each of the topics in this chapter.

Technological Advances

(1) *The Study of Gene Action,* by Bruce Wallace and Joseph Falkinham III. Ithaca: Cornell University Press (1997). This book describes recent methods used in the study of gene action. A companion volume of this book, dealing with the chemical nature of the gene, is *The Search for the Gene,* by Bruce Wallace. Ithaca: Cornell University Press (1992). (2) "DNA Chips: Promising

Toys Have Become Powerful Tools," by David Gerhold, Thomas Rushmore, and C. Thomas Caskey. *TIBS, 24:* 168–173 (1999).

Regulation

(*1*) "Eukaryotic Transcriptional Control," by Roger D. Kornberg. *TIBS, 24:* 46–49 (December 1999). (*2*) "Fundamentally Different Logic of Gene Regulation in Eukaryotes and Prokaryotes," by Kevin Struhl. *Cell, 98:* 1–4 (1999). (*3*) "Lac Repressor Map in Real Space," by Helen C. Pace, Michela A. Kercher, Ponzy Lu, Peter Markiewicz, Jeffrey H. Miller, Geoffrey Chang, and Mitchell Lewis. *TIBS, 22:* 334–339 (1997).

Development

(*1*) *The Making of a Fly: The Genetics of Animal Design,* by Peter Lawrence. Oxfords Blackwell Scientific (1992). (*2*) *Master Control Genes in Development of Evolution: The Homeobox Story,* by Walter J. Gering. New Haven: Yale University Press (1998).

Human Disease

(*1*) *Transcription Factors and Human Disease,* by Gregg L. Semenza. Oxford University Press (1998). (*2*) "The Hallmarks Of Cancer," by Douglas Hanahan and Robert A. Weinberg. *Cell, 100:* 57–70 (2000).

The Brain

Time, Love, Memory—A Great Biologist and His Quest for the Origins of Behavior, by Jonathan Weiner. New York: Alfred A. Knopf (1999). This is a biography of Seymour Benzer. An earlier review by Benzer is entitled: "Genetic Dissection of Behavior," in *Scientific American,* (December 1973: 24–39).

Recent papers from Benzer's laboratory:

1. *Spongecake* and *Eggroll,* Two Hereditary Diseases in *Drosophila* Resemble Patterns of Human Brain Degeneration," by Kyung-Tai Min and S. Benzer. *Current Biology, 7:* 885–888 (1997).
2. "Extended Lifespan and Stress Resistance in the *Drosophila* mutant *Methusala.* The Gene Encodes a Putative G-protein-coup Led Receptor," by Y.J. Lin, L. Seroude, and S. Benzer. *Science, 282:* 943–946 (1998).
3. "Preventing Neurodegeneration in the *Drosophila* mutant *Bubblegum,*" by K.T. Min and S. Benzer. *Science, 248:* 1986–1988 (1999).

INDEX